FINDING

CONNECTION

Shelter and Support for Parents of Children Living with
Mental Health and Neurodivergent Challenges

Janice Wiggins

A Mother on the Journey Sharing Her Realities

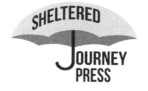

FIRST EDITION

Cover and Interior Design: Majid Khan
Development and Copy Editing: Cleo Miele

Sheltered Journey Press is an imprint of Sheltered Journey, Inc. www.shelteredjourney.org.

ISBN: 979-8-9918695-0-8 (print)
        979-8-9918695-1-5 (ebook)

Library of Congress Control Number: 2024926203

For my children, I love you.
(This mom thing isn't always pretty,
but I'm doing the very best I can and
learning every day.)

For parents on the journey,
may you feel acknowledged,
honored, and connected.

Try imagining a place where it's always safe and warm.

"Come in," she said,

"I'll give you shelter from the storm."

—Bob Dylan, "Shelter from the Storm"

CONTENTS

Introduction & How to Use This Book   1

Chapter 1   5

Finding Connection: The Power of Finding Someone Who "Gets It"

"While our realities as parents and caregivers of neurodiverse children vary, there are universal experiences that connect us."

Chapter 2   10

"Have You Tried . . . ?" Dealing with Helpful and Not-So-Helpful Advice Parents Receive

"Sometimes receiving unwanted and unsolicited advice aggravates, frustrates, and exhausts us much more than it helps."

Chapter 3 19

Relationships: How Our Connections Are Shaped by the Journey of Caring for a Child Living with Challenges

"It is hard to think of any relationships that are not in some way reshaped by the journey of parenting a child living with mental health and/or neurodivergent challenges."

Chapter 4 34

**Say It Again . . . and Again . . . and Again . . . :
Telling the Stories of the Journey**

"Sharing the stories, details, and experiences of a child's journey is often necessary to best advocate for them. However, in retelling and reliving this information, we can understandably grow tired and even forget the most painful details."

Chapter 5 44

The Blame Game: The Emotionally Exhausting Game of Finding Answers

"No one ever wins the blame game."

Chapter 6   55

The Forgotten Child: The Unique Challenges of the Siblings
of Children Living with Mental Health and Neurodivergent
Challenges

*"In moving heaven and earth for one child, the sibling(s) of that
child may feel overlooked and forgotten."*

Chapter 7   66

Medicated: The Issues and Biases of Psychiatric Medication

*"We all bring a lifetime of experiences and views on psychiatric
medication to the table when thinking about whether or not to
medicate."*

Chapter 8   80

The Things We Celebrate: Acknowledging and Honoring
Unique and Nontraditional Milestones of the Journey

*"As parents and caregivers of minor and adult children living with
challenges, our celebrations and special moments deserve to be
acknowledged, honored, and observed, no matter how small or
insignificant they may seem."*

Chapter 9   89

Punching Bag: When Parents Become Emotional Punching Bags

"It is common to feel like an emotional punching bag on the journey of loving and advocating for a child living with challenges."

Chapter 10   98

Surviving and Thriving: Living Fully While on the Journey

"There is a place somewhere between surviving and thriving where parents and caregivers of minor and adult children living with challenges can live, breathe, and grow."

Acknowledgments   107

Introduction

In April 2021, I started the *Sheltered Journey* podcast with the intention of sharing my journey of mothering a daughter living with emotional and developmental challenges and connecting with parents and caregivers on similar paths. Although I had regularly participated in and sometimes led support groups on the topic of parenting minor and adult children living with emotional, behavioral, developmental, and intellectual challenges, I thought a podcast would provide yet another way for parents and caregivers like me to feel less alone in the realness and rawness of the journey.

Sheltered Journey is my brutally honest account of the roller coaster ride of loving and advocating for my daughter. As I wrote and recorded episodes, I consciously focused on the common and extremely relevant issues, situations, and experiences on this journey that are often not talked about as a way to connect the huge and diverse community of parents and caregivers on this path. I also hoped the podcast would reveal these difficult realities to people who may not be on this particular journey with a child, but who want to learn, understand, and be more supportive of those in their lives who are.

The feedback to the podcast was overwhelmingly positive—parents reached out to tell me that listening made them feel less isolated, more understood, and that the podcast gave them a valuable support system. They told me that they laughed and cried as they realized that what they thought and felt were "unique" situations in their own lives were actually the shared experiences of many, many others. Some even said that they had encouraged family and friends to listen as a way of opening a dialogue with them about the realities of being on this path. Encouraged by this feedback, I continued doing episodes of the podcast—there are about forty-seven episodes to date—and started the Sheltered Journey nonprofit organization to further support parents and caregivers of minor and adult children living with mental health and neurodivergent challenges.

What I've learned from this process is that parents and caregivers of children living with challenges have a deep and profound need to be heard and understood not only by their family and friends, but also by health care professionals, school personnel, program administrators, and anyone else who is part of the system of care that supports their children. In order to achieve this understanding, we need to share the good, the bad, and the ugly parts of our stories without shame, blame, guilt, or fear of being misunderstood.

Finding Connection: Shelter and Support for Parents of Children Living with Mental Health and Neurodivergent Challenges builds on episodes of the Sheltered Journey podcast, with individual chapters devoted to common issues and experiences of parents and caregivers of children living with emotional, behavioral, developmental, and intellectual challenges. It is my hope that this book will provide even further connection and support for parents and caregivers on this journey as well as bring about understanding and compassion from those who want to support them.

How to Use This Book

Busy schedules and "to do" lists overwhelm most of our days, and my goal is that this book will not be another entry on a never-ending list of things to accomplish but rather a valuable resource we turn to when it is most needed. To that end, here are some ways to best fit this book into your life:

Read the chapters in whatever order you like. This book does not need to be read from beginning to end sequentially. Each chapter stands on its own, so you can easily pick the chapter(s) that best addresses what you are feeling or want to connect with and come back when you have the time and energy to read more.

Connect your personal experiences with the chapter subject. Each chapter ends with "For Further Thought" sections that encourage you to further connect with the content of a chapter.

Use individual chapters of the book to open a dialogue with family and friends. Sometimes the best way to share your experiences with others who may seem disconnected from or unaware of your reality is to have them read a chapter that illustrates what's happening in your life. Suggest a particular chapter for them to read, and then set up a time to talk about the chapter and how you relate to it.

Read the "Chapter Takeaways" when you don't have time to read a whole chapter but want to connect (or reconnect) to the subject. Sometimes we just don't have the time or energy to read an entire chapter—I get it! When that happens, take a peek at the "Chapter Takeaways" to get an overview and reminder of the subject matter.

Use the "Self-Care Workshop" sections to give yourself daily encouragement. "Self-Care Workshops" can be found at the end of each chapter and require just a few minutes to give yourself some much-needed time and attention.

It is my sincere hope that you find support, understanding, and compassion in the pages of this book. I wish you peace.

To listen to the Sheltered Journey podcast and learn more about the Sheltered Journey nonprofit organization, go to www.shelteredjourney.org.

Chapter 1

Finding Connection

The Power of Finding Someone Who "Gets It"

"While our realities as parents and caregivers of children living with mental health and neurodivergent challenges vary, there are universal experiences that connect us."

There is nothing quite like finding someone who "gets it." Someone who understands what you've been through and doesn't judge your feelings, reactions, and reality because they've been through something similar. Whenever I find someone who "gets" my reality, whatever that particular reality is, I feel a tremendous sense of relief and connection.

As the mother of a twenty-year-old daughter living with emotional and developmental challenges, I know what it is to yearn for someone who understands what it is like to be on this journey. Someone whom I can talk to openly and honestly about loving and advocating for my daughter and not sugarcoat the difficult experiences and feelings I have as a parent. Someone who understands the smallest of victories, the unlikeliest of celebrations, and shows compassion as I share my frustration, sadness, anger, resentment, and numbness sometimes toward my precious daughter as the result of being on this path for so many years. Someone who won't misunderstand, judge, or see me as a "bad parent" when they know my reality. In a nutshell, someone who just "gets it."

While our realities as parents and caregivers of minor and adult children living with mental health and neurodivergent challenges will vary, I have learned from my own experiences and those of close friends, from leading and participating in support groups, and from my work with the Sheltered Journey nonprofit organization that there are universal experiences that connect us.

It doesn't matter if you come from a large family or a small one. If you are a single parent, married, divorced, or widowed. If you are a birth parent or an adoptive parent. If you are a grandparent raising grandchildren or an aunt or uncle caring for nieces and nephews. It doesn't matter your age, race/ethnicity, political affiliation, or where you live. Sometimes, or much of the time, you may:

- Feel alone and isolated from friends and family because of a lack of understanding of the reality of your day-to-day life.

- Be overwhelmed and exhausted by the amount of people and systems you must deal with in order to best advocate for your child.

- Live with guilt and blame over your child's diagnosis and challenges.

- Struggle with the decision of whether or not to medicate your child or feel frustration that your minor or adult child refuses to take their prescribed medication.

- Get fed up with the amount of unwanted advice you receive from people who are "just trying to help."

- Feel as if you are an emotional and/or physical punching bag for your child's feelings and emotions.

- Have difficulty connecting to the love you have for your child because of years being on the never-ending roller coaster of emotions in caring and advocating for them.

- Wrestle with difficult emotions, such as anger, frustration, resentment, sadness, and hostility, directed toward your child.

- Worry about the effect this journey has on other relationships in your life—with your other children, spouses and romantic partners, extended family, and friendships.

- Feel anger and frustration at wanting to have just one day, one experience, one get-together without a meltdown or other disruptive behavior.

- Experience hopelessness as you wonder if things will ever get better.

- Feel guilty for taking care of yourself and living a full, rich life both despite and alongside your child's challenges.

I get what it feels like to have these feelings and emotions, because I've had similar ones myself.

It is my hope that, in addition to other parents on this path finding someone who "gets it" within these pages, this book will bring knowledge and understanding to people who may not be on this path with a child, but who want to learn, understand, and be more supportive of the people in their lives who are. One of the greatest gifts we can give each other as human beings is acceptance and understanding without judgment. In reading the stories, experiences, and vulnerabilities of parents and caregivers of children living with challenges, those unfamiliar with this journey can become better informed and able to provide compassionate, thoughtful support.

Regardless of the journey you are on, I hope you find connection within this book.

Chapter 1 Takeaways

• Finding connection with someone who "gets" your reality is invaluable.

• Although our journeys and realities are each different, parents and caregivers of children living with challenges share a wealth of common experiences and feelings.

For Further Thought

1. Have there been times in your life when you have connected with someone who truly understood and related to your experiences? If so, how did that connection make you feel? If not, what would you want someone to know about your reality so they could deeply connect with you?

2. If you could speak honestly (without fear of judgment) about your experiences in being the parent of a child living with challenges, what would you say?

Self-Care Workshop – Take Slow, Deep Breaths

Self-care can seem impossible at times, especially when so much of our life is devoted to caregiving. However, there are simple ways to take care of ourselves that we can build into each day. One powerful strategy is deep breathing.

Wherever you are—in the car, on the bus or train, in line at the supermarket, in a meeting, or even on the toilet (yep, sometimes the only place we can find peace is in the bathroom!)—take a few minutes to just breathe. Count to five as you breathe in through your nose, and then exhale through your mouth to the count of five. Do this simple exercise whenever you can to help lower your overall anxiety and improve your mood.

Chapter 2

"Have You Tried . . . ?"

Dealing with the Helpful and Not-So-Helpful Advice Parents Receive

---

"Sometimes receiving unwanted and unsolicited advice aggravates, frustrates, and exhausts us much more than it helps."

"Have you tried that series on Hulu about life in a Philadelphia public school? It's hilarious!"

"Have you tried taking the Garden State Parkway instead of the Turnpike? It's a prettier ride and you won't have all those eighteen-wheelers crowding you off the road."

"Have you tried the 'barnyard gravy' ice cream at the farmstead store out on Route 52? Sounds gross, but I guarantee you will love it!"

W e all give and receive "Have you tried . . . ?" advice and suggestions. Most people appreciate getting suggestions about television programs to watch, better routes to drive, ideas on where to find the best food, etc.

Parents and caregivers of children living with emotional, behavioral, developmental, and intellectual challenges receive *lots* of advice. Some of that advice comes from trained professionals who offer guidance that helps us better understand and support our child. Some of it comes from other parents who have been down a similar path, providing suggestions on how to better cope with our day-to-day realities.

However, we also receive loads of unwanted advice from family, friends, and even complete strangers who have no idea about or connection to our situations and circumstances or the issues involved in a particular diagnosis. Receiving "Have you tried . . . ?" advice and suggestions from these folks can aggravate, frustrate, and exhaust us much more than it helps us. And as a result of receiving so much unsolicited advice, we may even isolate ourselves from people and situations that bombard us with feedback because they are "just trying to help."

As the mother of a daughter living with emotional and developmental challenges, I have received endless unsolicited advice about ways to best care for and support my child. I've experienced multiple reactions to this unwanted advice:

- Sometimes after hearing such advice, I mumble to myself, "You have no (fill in your favorite expletive) clue," and walk away.

- Sometimes, I have a good ole ugly cry (to myself or to close friends who are aware of and understand the roller coaster journey of parenting a child living with challenges) and spit out some version of the following:

"Don't they realize I've already tried this and that a trillion times?"

"Do they have any idea of what a typical day is like? Let them come try it, then come back with that ridiculous (again, fill in your favorite expletive) advice."

"Do they have any idea how (expletive) exhausted I am and how hard I'm trying?"

• Sometimes I thank the person for their feedback, tell them that I appreciate their concern, and do my best to steer the conversation in a different direction.

• Sometimes I don't say anything, because I'm just too exhausted.

But as upset as I may get, I also realize there are times when I have been on the *giving* end of unwanted advice.

When I lived in New York City in early 2000, there was a woman about my age—I was thirty-six—whom I often saw around my East Side neighborhood. We'd bumped into each other plenty of times and traded enough pleasantries that I would call her a friendly acquaintance. I never knew her name, although I had spoken to her enough times that I probably should have, but it felt like we were so far into our "acquaintanceship" that it had become awkward to ask.

When I was about five months pregnant and heading home from a doctor's appointment, I ran into her as we waited for the crosstown bus. She congratulated me on my pregnancy—I was clearly showing—and asked how far along I was. I told her that I was in my second trimester and breathing a sigh of relief because my previous pregnancy had ended in a miscarriage in the first trimester, and I felt that I was out of the woods in terms of another miscarriage.

When she heard this, she said she understood the relief I felt and shared that she and her husband had experienced considerable trouble getting and staying pregnant and decided to stop trying. It was just too much heartache for them, she said.

When I heard this, I said—with way too much enthusiasm—that she had to go and see the fertility doctor I had seen, that this doctor accepted all major insurance plans, and that he was taking new patients. I also mentioned that there was a book another friend with fertility issues had suggested to me and that following the advice to the letter in this book definitely helped me get pregnant. I told the woman I was happy to lend her the book; I'd even highlight the most important information.

After I finished providing a torrent of "helpful" advice on what I considered to be the gold standard on conceiving—especially for women closing in on their fortieth birthday like we were—I noticed the woman's warm expression was replaced with a cold stare. Through clenched teeth, she mumbled:

"I said, we're done trying."

There was uncomfortable silence between us for several minutes. In truth, it felt like hours. Luckily, I could see the bus weaving through traffic as it made its way to our stop. We said a tense goodbye and got in line to board.

I felt horrible after that exchange. All I had wanted to do was help, and I thought she would be receptive because I didn't mean any harm—yet the advice I offered had caused harm. A few months after my first child was born, my husband and I moved out of the city to the suburbs and I never saw the woman again.

Every time I think of that conversation, I cringe. Especially because on the journey of loving and advocating for a child living with challenges, I truly realize how it feels to receive advice, suggestions, emails with links to articles "I just have to read," etc. from well-meaning people who don't have a clue as to everything that's been tried, every professional who's been seen, every research article that's been read, every Google search that's been done, every YouTube video that's been watched, and every approach that's been tried and retried.

I'm not saying that I know everything about my daughter's diagnoses and challenges. However, I am saying, asking, wishing, and pleading for those wanting to offer advice to tread lightly and consider that the advice they offer often falls upon ears that have received plenty of unwanted advice.

Yet, despite everything I've said here about unsolicited advice and how it can be difficult to receive, it's a slippery slope to navigate. Sometimes advice we didn't ask for can help. For example, I learned about my daughter's therapeutic school from a conversation I had with another mother who told me I should look into the school she sent her son to because it offered a level of psychiatric support—psychiatrists on duty, daily group sessions, weekly therapy, and family support sessions—unlike any other school in our area. I hadn't asked to hear about the school, but I thank God she told me about it. V attended the school for several years, and it helped her (and me) tremendously.

But there are plenty of times when I have to say, "Hold the advice." For example, when someone told me that there was a woman who lived in another country and if I could scrape together enough money to fly V over to see this shaman-type woman, V would be "cured." Apparently, being in the presence of this magical woman would somehow help V. This was wildly outlandish advice, at least to me, but the person who offered it was so sincere, so well-meaning, that I gritted my teeth, squeezed out a smile, and said:

"Thanks for the suggestion."

Consider the advice other parents of children living with challenges have shared with me. Advice to:

Change their child's diet, because if they do that, then the diagnosis will be different.

Read about a case—albeit a highly unusual and unlikely one—where someone with a similar diagnosis as their child suddenly began speaking when they had never spoken before.

Love their child more, because that would solve everything. (As if the parent didn't already love her son with every atom of her body.)

Advice to be tougher, softer, stricter, nicer, more or less accommodating. Advice to try harder, to worry less or worry more.

Some of the hardest "Have you tried . . . ?" statements can come from parents and caregivers on similar paths as ours. I once attended a support group with the parent of a child who was newly diagnosed. This parent was a fountain of advice, eagerly offering up advice to a more seasoned parent whose child had the same diagnosis, but this parent's child was several years older and took more of a "been there,

15

done that" kind of attitude in response. With every suggestion offered to the more seasoned parent, I could see how she tensed up and said (more like growled) things like, "Yes, we've already tried that," and then withdrew from the conversation altogether.

When offering advice to parents and caregivers of children living with challenges, sensitivity is key. Think of "Have you tried . . . ?" statements and advice like you would a traffic light. If someone clearly asks you for advice or suggestions in regard to their child, you are at a green light, and you can move forward with your feedback.

In any other situation where you are not being asked for advice, consider yourself at a yellow light and proceed with caution, or maybe even at a red light where you stop with the dispensing of advice completely. Odds are, it's not wanted.

When the woman from my old neighborhood told me that she and her husband had stopped trying to conceive because there was just too much heartache in the process, *that was my red light, and I should have stopped.* When I think back to the woman's situation, undoubtedly she had been pummeled with well-meaning advice many times before and had constructed a well-worn defense system for every time someone offered a "magic solution" to her fertility issues. Instead of speeding through her red light, I could have said something as simple as "I get that," "I understand," or "That must have been difficult." That's all that was needed. It wasn't my place to solve this woman's situation; I just needed to acknowledge the words she said and move on. Period.

I realize that "Have you tried . . . ?" advice most often comes from a good place and a desire to resolve an issue, relieve someone's pain, or make things better in some way. But sometimes that advice isn't helpful, and it can cause frustration and emotional pain rather than relief. If you are the parent or caregiver of a child living with challenges, you more than likely have been on the receiving end of lots of advice—some helpful, some not. The ways we react to advice that is not helpful will be different depending on who we are and the particular situation or circumstance we find ourselves in. However, here are some ideas you might consider:

Acknowledge the advice and change the subject. In this case, you respond with a simple "Thank you for the advice" (or something to that effect) and then change the subject by saying something like, "Tell me about how you have been doing," or "How's it going with . . . ?" One thing I know for sure is that most people love talking about themselves, so diverting the conversation away from you and onto them tends to work well.

Acknowledge the advice, but refuse to talk about it. Similar to the previous advice, you can say, "Thanks for the feedback," but instead of diverting the conversation, you then shut it down entirely by saying you don't want to talk further about your child and/or the situation. You might say something like: "I don't want to discuss this now," "Now is not the time," or "I'm overwhelmed right now and would prefer not to talk about it."

Acknowledge and explain that you are aware and on top of the situation. Here, you would say something like: "Thank you for the advice. I/we are well aware of the situation and are handling it."

Receiving advice—both wanted and unwanted—is an unavoidable part of life, and certainly a significant part of parenting a child living with challenges. No matter which way you respond to unwanted advice, always remember that as a parent, you are doing the very best you can with the resources you have.

Chapter 2 Takeaways

- Parents and caregivers receive lots of advice and suggestions on ways to best take care of their children. Some of this advice can be more frustrating than helpful.

- There are several ways to address unwanted feedback, such as changing the subject, refusing to talk about it, or firmly stating that you are already handling the situation.

For Further Thought

1. What advice have you received in regard to your child, and how did you respond?

2. What type of response would you like to give (that you haven't tried in the past) to someone who offers you unwanted advice?

Self-Care Workshop – Dream a Little Dream

Daydreaming can be a powerful escape that adds to our well-being. We might, for example, recall a time in our life that brought us peace, passion, joy, or uncontrollable belly laughs. Take a few minutes out of your day to dream; enjoy the momentary respite.

Chapter 3

Relationships

How Our Connections Are Shaped by the Journey of Caring for a Child Living with Challenges

---

"It is hard to think of any relationships that are not in some way reshaped by the journey of parenting a child living with mental health and/or neurodiverse challenges."

Here's a question for you to consider: How does having a minor or adult child living with emotional, behavioral, developmental, or intellectual challenges affect the relationships in your life, both positively and negatively? Think about it for a moment.

In my twenty-plus years of being V's mother, I cannot think of one significant relationship in my life that has not in some way been affected by this journey. Some of my relationships have ended, and some have grown. Some have become a source of frustration and anger, while others have added a calming presence to my life. And while I can't speak for every parent, I think it's safe to say that many have seen their relationships change shape in one way or another on this path.

For example, when participating in and leading support groups and interacting with other parents and caregivers, I notice one topic comes up often: relationships.

Relationships with our children, with our friends, with our spouses and romantic partners, with our close and extended family; with people involved in our child's care; with work colleagues; with neighbors; and, the most important relationship, with ourselves.

I listen to parents talk about close friendships that are no longer supportive after the diagnosis of a child, marriages and romantic partnerships shaken by the realities of caring for a child with mental illness, or extended family connections strained by outside judgment and misunderstanding. Parents and caregivers beating themselves up over decisions they made or didn't make.

Let's take a closer look at some of the relationships in our lives and how they are shaped and reshaped by the experiences and circumstances of this journey.

Relationships with Our Children

Certainly, the relationship we have with our children—whether neurodivergent or neurotypical, whether they live with or without mental health challenges—is affected on this path. Any parent-child relationship has its ups and downs; that's a given. But when you mix in the realities, complexities, and impossible situations that occur on this journey, resentment, anger, exhaustion, fear, and a bunch of other difficult emotions can take root.

The relationship I have with my daughter, V—who lives with neurological and mental health challenges—encompasses a roller coaster of emotional highs and lows. One of the most difficult parts of this relationship is that I often feel disconnected from the abundant love I have for her. It's still there, but after so many years on this journey, I can't tap into it in the way I would like to; sometimes I just feel "numb" toward her. It has taken me a long time to admit this to myself, and I feel a great deal of shame over it, but that is my reality and I own it.

As a way to explain this numbness, both to myself and other people I've talked to on this journey, I think of Niagara Falls. The Falls are alive—powerful, vibrant, and abundant. But with frigidly cold temperatures, the mist and spray form a thick crust of ice over top of the rushing water, making it appear as if the Falls are completely frozen. Yet, water continues to flow underneath the sheets of ice. The water never stops flowing; it is always there and always moving.

Like Niagara Falls, my love for V is bold and abundant. It never stops flowing, but due to a complex mixture of difficult situations and realities, it sometimes freezes up and grows numb. As a mother, I feel ashamed sharing all of this because when we think of a mother's emotions toward her children, the word "numb" isn't usually an acceptable adjective. However, this is a reality that was cathartic for me to admit.

And what about our relationships with the siblings of our child living with challenges? My relationship with M, V's older sister, has been strained at times because M feels that I pay so much attention to everything that goes into helping V live her best life that her own needs are sometimes ignored. These feelings M has of being overlooked and pushed to the side to make room for V and her needs is a common one for siblings of children living with mental health and neurological challenges. (In chapter six of this book, titled "The Forgotten Child," I talk more about my relationship with M and sibling relationships in general.)

With the help of lots of therapy (for her and for me), time, and difficult conversations between us in which I put my ego aside and listen to, acknowledge, and honor her feelings, my connection with M is healing. But I accept that there may always be an undercurrent within M of feeling like she's "the one left out" that is a part of my relationship with her.

As a parent or caregiver on this path, our relationships with our children can sometimes be a knotted mess. Our feelings toward them may run from hot to cold in a given day—maybe within an hour. Numbness may have worked its way into your heart as it did mine. I am doing the best I can with my children, and that's all that I can do. Are there things I miss? Yes. Are there mistakes I make? Yes. But I serve no one by beating up on myself over the relationships I have with my children, and neither do you.

In terms of the relationships we have with our children, we can only try to learn, grow, and move forward.

Relationships with Our Spouses and Romantic Partners

One type of relationship that goes through all sorts of changes on this journey is the one we share with a husband, wife, or romantic partner. On their own, these relationships will naturally have their ups and downs, and that's to be expected when two individuals come together and decide to share their lives.

Having children certainly affects these relationships, but when you mix in a child who lives with additional challenges, some of these relationships find themselves on shaky ground. Those relationships are then reshaped and redefined, both positively and negatively.

There are many reasons for this, especially since every relationship and person is different. However, I can only speak from my own experiences, and what I've learned from interacting with many other parents on this path. So, why does this happen?

From my sixteen-year marriage—and I would say this is fairly common in any partnership—having an uneven balance of responsibilities in caring for my daughter V gradually chipped away at the foundation of our union.

Sometimes one person in a couple—and very often that person is the mother, though it can certainly be either partner—handles what feels like everything in the support and advocacy of a child. She takes the phone calls from school and talks to the teachers, nurses, social workers, psychologists, and other school personnel. She fills out countless forms and communicates with case managers. She calls in the crisis team and sometimes the police, talks to speech and occupational therapists, psychiatrists, pediatricians, neurologists, and any other practitioners involved in her child's care. She keeps the schedule, holds on to records, and monitors medications. She answers the questions about her child that are almost always directed at her, argues with the insurance companies, and spends countless hours trying to figure out how to work within the system in order to get the best care for her child.

And that's just for one child. What about any other children in the family—children with or without challenges? Most often, it is one parent more than the other attending to their needs, meaning that one person's plate in the couple is always full to overflowing. Thus, that person's tank teeters on empty most days.

For me, having such an imbalance for many years led to what felt like an unshakeable resentment toward my husband. Was that the reason our marriage ultimately ended? No. There were many other reasons. And I will also say, in my ex-husband's defense, that I could have loosened up my grip of control over every aspect of V's care and let him help more. Nevertheless, when there is such an imbalance, marriages and romantic partnerships can suffer.

Another issue that may form between partners or spouses is recognition of a child's challenges and finding agreement on the best way to handle these challenges.

I noticed very early in V's life that there were differences in her development compared to that of her older sister. When V began preschool, those differences became more pronounced, and I often heard from teachers that she was struggling emotionally in class and had trouble with comprehension. The summer before entering kindergarten, with the encouragement of a very astute preschool teacher, I had V evaluated by our school district and she received an Individualized Education Program (IEP). With an IEP, V would receive specialized instruction and related services that were tailored to her particular emotional and learning challenges.

My ex-husband is and continues to be deeply devoted to both of our children, and he loves them unconditionally, but our marriage was strained by the disagreements we had in acknowledging V's struggles and the best ways to address them. I talked with him often about my concerns (and the concerns of V's preschool teachers), but after being met with endless versions of denial and urgings to "just give her time and she'll be fine," I went through with the necessary intervention strategies pretty much on my own. Unsurprisingly, this created distance between us and further bruised our relationship.

Although this wasn't a major issue in my marriage, I've heard from other parents that they often become the receiver of their partner's anger, resentment, and blame over issues connected to their child's mental health and neurological challenges. In these troublesome situations, parents may become enemies.

I wish I could offer some easy answers to these marriage and partnership issues, but none exist. I do think, however, that couple's therapy can be a great asset. My former husband and I were in couple's therapy for over two years, and although our marriage eventually ended—because, as I said earlier, there were many other issues involved in our split—talking with him each week with the support of a therapist helped us better communicate our concerns, needs, and struggles in connection with both of our children. Really, even the most solid of marriages and partnerships can benefit from therapeutic support when dealing with the realities of supporting children with mental health and neurological challenges.

In addition, I want to say a few words for those of us, myself included, who are not currently in relationships but hope to find one that is healthy, nurturing, and supportive.

I've been divorced for several years now, dated my fair share, and had short-lived relationships since then, but none that stuck. Sometimes I wonder why I continue to search—maybe it's all the sappy love stories I read about and see in movies. Maybe it's seeing couples in my life who are in healthy, loving relationships and wanting that in my own life. Maybe it's hearing about three of my dear friends who found love late in life. Whatever the reason, I remain open.

Yet despite this openness, there's an interesting wrinkle that comes up for parents and caregivers on this journey who are searching for love. I have been on all of the major dating apps (yes, I'll admit it), and one common line that I see stated in different ways is "I want a partner with NO drama."

How does a parent on this journey respond to someone who says, "I don't want to deal with drama!"? Beats me, because if a prospective date reads this book or learns anything about me from a virtual search, they'll quickly find out that my life has drama. But here's the catch: Just because there is drama in my life in no way means that I will bring that drama to a partner. Perhaps this is better understood by someone who is on this path or at least empathetic to it.

Relationships with Extended Family

Relationships with our extended family—our parents, grandparents, siblings, nieces/nephews, cousins, aunties, uncles, etc.—are sometimes also shaped by this journey.

In a perfect world, these relationships would always be supportive, especially when it comes to having a child living with challenges. But the world we live in is far from perfect, and as a result, our relationships with extended family can be taxing.

I have a small extended family—I often joke that we could have Thanksgiving dinner in a Volkswagen Beetle. We talk on occasion, but I wouldn't say that we are particularly close. As a result, they don't play a significant role in my life.

However, that is not the case for many parents on this journey. Sometimes we have relatives who offer loving support and step in to help whenever they can—what a blessing! But sometimes, our relatives are judgmental of our decisions and lack understanding of our day-to-day realities. These relatives may not be able to comprehend why we never invite them over. While the reasons for this are many, sometimes the reason is simply that our homes are in such disarray, we are embarrassed to reveal what our "everyday" home looks like.

I have a friend on this journey whose son regularly punches holes in the walls of her home, destroys family photos and other art hung on the wall, and tears apart books and newspapers left out. She has told me that she dreads having anyone over because her house always feels "upside-down." Relatives sometimes don't understand why we can't make solid plans for an outing and don't get that we don't always know what state our child will be in on that particular day, so can't make a plan concrete. Sometimes they criticize our parental techniques and offer advice and suggestions we didn't ask for—see chapter 2 of this book, titled "Have You Tried . . . ?"

You can try to talk to your family and explain your reality, of course. Sometimes that will be met with understanding and empathy; sometimes it will not. If a relative plays a significant role in your and your child's life, you might consider inviting them to a family session with a therapist if that is a possibility. You may even try to educate a relative on some of the realities of this journey by sharing this book with them (and referring them to a specific chapter(s) that can add to their understanding of parts of your life).

Relationships with Friends

Friendships are an important part of our lives, and good friends— people who are supportive, understanding, and want the very best for us—are worth their weight in gold. Many of us on this journey have experienced friendships that have either blossomed, strengthened, stagnated, or faded away, because in caring for a child living with challenges, what we need from our friends changes as well.

For me, any free time that I have outside of working and caring for my family is mostly spent with people who know of, understand, or have some connection to the realities of parenting a child living with challenges. It's not that I don't love and appreciate all of my friends, but as a result of being on this path, I now speak a different language. This language—one of exhaustion, anger, frustration, hopelessness, and fear of the unknown and all its diagnosis-specific dialects—is understood by others on this journey, but not necessarily by people who have no connection to it. And most times, I simply don't have the energy to translate.

Parents have told me numerous stories about once-close friendships that:

• Became tense because of the amount of unwanted advice and suggestions coming from friends who knew nothing about their child's diagnosis and all that is involved.

• Grew distant because a friend didn't understand why they never had time or energy to go places and do the things they used to.

• Faded away because a friend didn't understand why they suddenly had to change plans or leave things open because of their child's shifting emotions and behavior.

I've also heard stories of friends who, not knowing what to say or do, simply disappeared. But our friendships are also capable of growing and adjusting to this new reality. There are many such stories.

I was once visiting a friend who, after many tumultuous days, had taken her daughter to the emergency room to get a psychiatric evaluation. I offered to bring food or check in on her other daughter who was at home, but she said a different friend who lived in the area had it covered. She didn't know how long she would be in the ER with her daughter, but that friend was going to make sure she was fed and that her daughter at home was taken care of. This kind of friendship is truly priceless.

My closest and dearest friend and I agreed to never pressure or make each other feel guilty about phone calls, whether it be making them or calling back. We understand that our friendship is not defined by who calls the most or who sent the last text. Having such an agreement has given me peace and relief from feeling as if I'm a "bad friend" or that I'm not holding up my end of the friendship when in reality, I just don't have the time or energy to reach out or stay connected.

I hope that everyone has a friend (or friends) that gives more than they take and understands when others don't. If you don't have friends who understand your journey, I have found that parent/caregiver support groups can help provide that connection. To find a support group in your area, go to shelteredjourney.org and look up resources in your state.

The Relationship with Ourselves

Lastly, we must consider the relationship we have with ourselves. This one is rarely simple and is most certainly complicated by all of the experiences, incidents, and events we have accumulated from our own childhood until now. Having a child living with challenges can make that relationship more complex—while any caregiver can lose themselves in the process of caring for someone else, when you add in the complexities of caring for a child with mental health or neurodivergent challenges specifically, that connection to ourselves can seem even harder to reach.

As much as we may overlook or minimize it, this relationship is, in fact, the most important one in our lives, because it affects our mental and physical health and serves as the foundation for all of our other relationships.

It has taken me many years to realize the importance of having a healthy relationship with myself. At times, it is a struggle to have such a relationship, because it seems more natural to beat myself up over every negative incident or event in my life rather than show myself compassion, grace, and a willingness to learn from both the good and not-so-good things that happen.

With that said, I know my relationship with V is very much shaped by how well (or not well) I take care of myself. If, for example, I have had a good night's sleep, take some time to read, do a crossword puzzle or some other brain game, and exercise my body, I am much better able to withstand and ride the inevitable wave of emotions in our relationship. When I regularly see a therapist to better understand and work on myself, my relationship with V—and all the other relationships in my life—benefits.

I will always need to work on maintaining a healthy relationship with myself so that I can be my own best advocate and friend, and I don't think I'm alone in this. So many of the people in my life struggle with having a healthy relationship with themselves; it seems to be a constant journey. Thankfully, there are many different ways to build a healthier relationship with ourselves. While some strategies may work for some and not others, here are a few that you might find helpful:

Set aside time just for yourself. This is definitely easier said than done, as sometimes it might seem like the only time we have for ourselves is when we're in the bathroom! (I definitely remember feeling this way when my daughters were very young.) In that lengthy "to do" list of yours, carve out a few minutes each day just for you; you might even set an alarm that reminds you to take a break for some "me time." Sit down with a cup of tea, listen to one of your favorite songs, or just daydream. That's right, daydream about a particularly pleasurable experience in your life. (That one's a favorite of mine.)

Consider seeing a therapist. If you know me well, you likely know that I am a huge advocate of individual therapy. I sometimes joke that if I were president of the United States, I would require individual therapy for everyone at various points of their lives! (Grandiose, I know, but I think self-reflection is invaluable.) Therapy can provide you with better and stronger coping strategies, greater self-awareness, and stress relief. Finding a therapist—either in person or virtually— might be something to explore if you haven't done so already.

Take an electronics break. Even if just for a few minutes, put away all your electronics and give yourself a moment to take a few deep breaths and pay attention to your surroundings without the ring or ping of a cellphone, laptop, tablet, smartwatch, or any other electronic device.

Surround yourself with positive affirmations. I'm a big fan of positive affirmations—those statements that bring about positive thinking and can help reframe negative thoughts. Sometimes they stick with me and sometimes they don't, but I find that if I have them in front of me every day, they make a difference. For example, I have a fairly large sign in a central location of my living room that reads: "Do one thing every day that makes you happy." Because this sign is in such a prominent place, this forces me to at least think about this affirmation and—hopefully—follow through and do something to bring myself joy.

Take a walk. No matter my mood, I find a sense of peace when I take a walk, whether it be a brief walk around the corner with my dog or something longer when I'm alone. Movement can make a huge difference in our mindset.

Celebrate your victories, even the smallest ones. It may seem easier to celebrate others in your life, but be sure to congratulate yourself on your victories, too—both big and small. For example, I congratulate myself when I get to bed on time. While that may seem small, to me it's huge because I know I'm getting the much-needed rest I need.

Of all of the relationships we will ever have in our lives, the one with ourselves is key. Do what you can to consistently develop and work on having a healthy relationship with yourself.

We have many relationships in our lives, and those connections can and likely will be affected by the realities of having a child living with challenges. Some of these relationships will feel easy, and some will not. Some will bring joy, and some will not. Some can be healed, and some cannot. And inevitably, that's life, right? I wish there were magic solutions to healing all of the relationships in our lives, but none exist. I do think, however, that simply acknowledging the ways in which relationships in our lives can be reshaped by being on this journey can help us to better understand them.

No matter the state of the relationships in your life—with your children, spouses and romantic partners, extended family, friendships, and even with yourself—I wish you peace.

Chapter 3 Takeaways

- The relationships in our life—with our children, friends, spouses or romantic partners, extended family, etc.—are often affected by the realities of caring for a child living with challenges.

- The relationship we have with ourselves is the most important one in our lives, as it affects our mental and physical health and serves as the foundation for all of our other relationships.

For Further Thought

1. How have the relationships in your life changed (positively, negatively, or not at all) since being on this journey?

2. What are some changes you would like to see in your various relationships?

3. What are some ways that you can build a healthier relationship with yourself?

Self-Care Workshop – Start a Gratitude Practice

Think of something you are grateful for. It doesn't have to be anything major—just an ordinary event that somehow enhanced your day. The key to practicing gratitude is focusing on small things rather than big ones. Did you enjoy a cup of coffee or tea, avoid traffic on your way to school, notice the beauty of the sun, or find shelter from a rainstorm today? All of these are things to notice and be grateful for, and expressing that gratitude can add to your sense of well-being.

Chapter 4

Say It Again . . . and Again . . . and Again . . .

Telling the Stories of the Journey

"Sharing the stories, details, and experiences of a child's journey is often necessary to best advocate for them. However, in retelling and reliving this information over and over again, we can understandably grow tired and even forget the most painful details."

D o you remember those pull-string talking dolls from the 1960s and 70s? You'd pull a plastic ring attached to a string at the back of the doll and it would utter a few standard phrases. With one pull, you might hear Chatty Cathy—the first of these dolls—say, "I love you," "I hurt myself," or "May I have a cookie?" in a childlike singsong voice. I was transfixed when my parents bought me one of those dolls for my fifth birthday. I'd sit in the corner of the room I shared with my sister and yank the string so many times that the plastic ring eventually fell off.

I sometimes feel like a human version of one of those pull-string dolls whenever I share some part of my daughter V's mental health journey. Last month, we visited her psychiatrist. V had seen this psychiatrist before (she'd worked at the therapeutic school V attended), but V had since graduated and the psychiatrist no longer worked at the school. Since she had no access to V's records, we needed to start from scratch. So, for what felt like the 999th time, I explained V's journey to someone in need of details, something like a Chatty Cathy doll:

Doctor: (pulls the imaginary string attached to my back and asks): "When did V first start seeing a therapist?"

Me: (reciting the answer as the string slowly recoils): "She was around five, just before starting kindergarten."

Doctor: (pulls string again): "How old was V when she started medication?"

Me: (reciting a short answer as the string snaps back): "I think it was around nine or ten."

And then this back-and-forth question-and-answer session continued on as it always does:

- Has she been hospitalized? How many times? Where and when?
- Has she been to outpatient programs? Which ones and when?
- Residential placements? Where, when, and for how long?
- What medications is she taking now? What's the dosage for each?

In the early days of our journey before V had an actual diagnosis (and when her epic meltdowns drilled into every nook and cranny of our lives), the story I was most often asked to tell—by the pediatrician,

35

neurologist, therapist, school social worker, etc.—was V's birth story:

Forty-one weeks . . . midwife in hospital . . . doctors called in . . . cord wrapped around neck twice . . . definitely should have been a C-section, but it was too late . . . hole in heart but healed up on its own . . . she seemed fine, but I noticed differences between her and her older sister when she was around eighteen months . . . yada, yada, yada . . .

As the years pass, I keep adding chapters to the story and reciting the details when needed.

A friend of mine also on this journey keeps a timeline of her daughter's mental health history so that she can easily recite the necessary details whenever she needs to just by pulling up a file on her laptop. That makes a lot of sense, and it would save me from having to dig through my memories to reconstruct specific details that I've wanted to forget or going through file folders stuffed with medical records, psychiatric evaluations, IEPs, neurological reports, etc. But to be honest, it's too difficult, too emotional, too raw for me to put together such a timeline. So, for now at least, I just answer the questions again and again, piecing together the details of the story as best I can.

Like me, parents and caregivers of children living with challenges may feel like some version of a pull-string doll when they have to recite stories, details, and experiences to medical professionals, school personnel, relatives, friends, bosses/work colleagues, neighbors, etc. And while we share pieces of our child's journey often, the details don't fall from our lips in the leisurely, lighthearted way a fictional bedtime story is read to a child or how tall tales about an eccentric uncle are passed down from generation to generation at the Thanksgiving Day dinner table.

When we tell these stories over and over again, we relive the pain of what happened, feel the frustration and fear of what could have happened, and experience anew the sadness and isolation that comes with the reality of the story.

And yet, we must share these stories so that we get our child much-needed therapeutic support, services, and hopefully, understanding.

I once had to repeatedly tell a particularly difficult story about a situation involving twelve-year-old V. (We're going to need to pull the imaginary string attached to my back about a mile long and let it slooooowly recoil for this one . . .)

I'd gone out on a date (because hey, in addition to being the mother of two children, I am also a divorced middle-aged woman trying to construct some kind of life for myself, although I haven't been very successful at it). Anyway, about forty minutes into the date, I get a call from V's older sister, M (whom I'd left in charge), saying that I needed to come home right away. There had been an incident between V and a boy who should not have been at my house at the time. (V had conveniently waited until I left to invite the boy over.)

When I got home—I'd only been ten minutes away—police cruisers were parked outside. Inside, four officers stood in the living room while V hysterically clutched onto my ex-husband. (My oldest daughter had also called my ex, who lives close by.)

I won't get into the details of this story; I'll just sum it up by saying a tough yet friendly female officer covered in tattoos and her partner stayed behind to take down the necessary information for the police report (the other two officers left shortly after I arrived), there was a search for the boy involved, a detective was put on the case, and the case was later assigned to the district attorney's office.

I'm not sharing the specific details of this story because that's not the point. The point is that this particular incident, this story, had to be repeated to multiple people multiple times, and telling various versions of it felt like a punch to the gut every time I told it.

I first attempted to tell my date what I thought might be going on at home and why I had to leave so abruptly. I tried to explain it to him and include all the relevant details I'd grown used to repeating:

"A . . . D . . . XYZ."

And I gotta say, this guy should have been called "The Flash," because after my short explanation he got up and went to the door of the restaurant so fast, his disappearance rivaled the speed of any comic book superhero—now you see him, now you don't.

After the police left our house and I settled V down, I continued telling the story, this time to my next-door neighbors who are close friends and grew concerned when they saw police cruisers parked outside my house. So, I told them the story based on what I knew:

"ABC," then "DEFG," then "HIJKLMNOPQRSTUVWXYZ."

I thanked my neighbors for their concern and went back into the house.

I then left a message for V's case manager, the person who coordinates V's various services. I wanted to tell the story while it was fresh in my mind, not wait until the morning when the details might get diluted by the events of a new day. So, here we go again:

"Hi, it's Janice Wiggins. Something happened tonight involving V

and I wanted to keep you in the loop. ABC, DEF, GHIJK, LMNO, P, QR, STUV, WXYZ. Please call me as soon as you can."

I have learned that when you are telling the story to people who are directly in charge of your child's services—sometimes a whole team of people—you need to tell the story clearly, thoroughly, and as accurately as possible, even if you don't want to remember it clearly, thoroughly, or accurately, so that the story is documented and necessary services are provided. Even if you would much rather forget the whole damn thing happened at all.

A good friend called that same night to see how the date went. I then told the story again, but this time I was brief:

"ABC, WXYZ."

My friend knows our journey; she didn't need additional details.

The next morning, I called V's school therapist to tell her the story. (V attends a therapeutic school for children with significant emotional and psychiatric challenges.)

"ABCDEFGHIJKLMNOPQRSTUVWXYZ."

V's therapist thought I should also speak to her psychiatrist, given V's impulsive behavior increasing in frequency in the past several weeks; maybe an adjustment in medication needed to be considered. So, I spoke to the psychiatrist a little later in the day.

"Hello, doctor. Well, ABC . . . DEF . . . GHI . . . JKL, MNOPQ . . . RSTUVWXYZ."

After my talk with the psychiatrist, my ex-husband called to see where things stood:

"ABCDEFGHIJKLMNOPQRSTUVWXYZ. Sorry if I'm being short with you, but I'm tired of talking about it."

Given what happened, I took V to the pediatrician to be examined and told the story again:

"ABCDEFGHI . . . JKLMNO . . . PQRSTUVWXYZ."

On the way home, I remembered that I needed to contact V's behavioral therapist so that she knew the story too:

"ABCDEFG, HIJKLMNOPQRSTUVWXYZ."

Later—I can't remember what day this was—I went to the police station to get an update on the case. The detective assigned to the case wasn't in, but another detective was there, and I told him the story in the hopes he could dig up some information and share it with me.

"ABCDEFGHIJKLMNOPQRSTUVWXYZ."

He was friendly and patiently listened to my telling of the story, but he couldn't give me any additional information. I needed to wait for the detective in charge of the case to get back to me.

My mother called to check in. She was in her early eighties at the time and definitely didn't need to hear the story.

"How's everything?" my mom asked.

"We're hanging in, Mom," I replied; there was no need to upset her.

Then there was another member of V's team who wasn't in regular contact but still needed to be kept in the loop for when she saw V again, and so I called her to tell the shortened version of the story:

"ABC, WXYZ. Just wanted to let you know. Call me if you have questions."

A freelance project I had been working on would be delayed because I'd been overwhelmed (much more so than I normally am), so I told the story to the project supervisor:

"ABC . . . XYZ."

She only needed to know the outline of the story and why I'd miss the deadline, not the details. Besides, I felt too scared to tell her anything more because she might think I was too worn out and refuse to send me any additional projects (and I desperately needed the work).

So, did you happen to count the number of times I told this particular story, both in full and abbreviated versions? Let's see: there was the date (aka "The Flash"), the neighbors, the friend, the case manager, the therapist, the psychiatrist, the ex-husband, the pediatrician, the behavioral therapist, the detective, my mother, the work supervisor . . .

But you know what? It doesn't really matter how many times it was, because even telling the story once is too many.

I realize that it is necessary to tell the stories, to share the details and experiences because it is all part of being on the front lines of advocating for our children. Perhaps all the stories are not as dramatic as the one I just told, but they are still a regular part of our lives and need to be recited when we see a new doctor or a new therapist, enter a new program, talk to a school counselor, share with family and friends not familiar with our story, move to a new city or state—whenever we need to fill in the blanks of our child's journey.

And when we grow tired of telling the story, it is for good reason. When we sometimes forget the most painful details of the story, it is understandable. And when we feel that we can't tell the story anymore, yet somehow we do, we should give ourselves grace.

I don't know what your stories are, but I am sure you have plenty of them and may feel like a pull-string doll as you answer the questions and recite the details yet again. I get it, and I understand the agony, anger, frustration, fear, impatience, embarrassment, and everything else you may feel in telling the story.

I also realize that keeping the details of V's story in my head is not ideal, and I am working on better ways to capture her journey despite the mental block I often encounter when I have to remember. I suggest keeping track of the details of your child's histories on a computer, as my friend does. Or, instead of typing and saving the details in a file on your computer, you may just keep notes on your smartphone or speak the details of the story into an audio recording on your phone that you can refer back to at a later date.

Whatever your stories are, I understand that they may be difficult to recall and retell, and I wish you peace in the process of retelling and reliving them.

Chapter 4 Takeaways

- Parents can easily become overwhelmed and exhausted by the continuous explaining of details and experiences involved with their child's care.

- Repeatedly telling the same story feels like reliving it over and over again.

For Further Thought

1. What have been your experiences in sharing the details of your child's story?

2. How does telling the story multiple times to multiple different people affect you?

3. How do you keep track of the details of the story? Can you think of any alternative ways to help you better keep track?

Self-Care Workshop – Display Positive Affirmations

Positive affirmations are short phrases or statements that can help you focus on what's most important in your life, build your self-esteem and confidence, and provide you with a healthy outlook on life. You can come up with your own affirmations or look online for ideas (Google "positive affirmations" and you'll find plenty!). Here's one that I often say to myself:

"It ain't pretty, but I did it and that's all that matters." I like this saying because it reminds me to take risks and get things done, even if they don't go exactly as I planned.

Once you've come up with some favorite affirmations, print them out or write them down and put them in places where you can easily see them every day, like on your nightstand, your car dashboard, your laptop, or the home screen of your smartphone.

Chapter 5

The Blame Game

The Emotionally Exhausting Game of Finding Answers

"No one ever wins the blame game."

A t one time or another, we all play the "blame game." I'll get into more detail about this in a bit, but in a nutshell, the blame game involves blaming yourself (and sometimes others) for painful experiences, situations, and events in your life.

I've been playing this game for most of my life, but I became an expert at it when I was around nine years old and my parents split up. My version of the blame game involved blaming myself for my dad building a new family while erasing any trace of me and my sister from his life. To my preadolescent self, it was surely my fault. I was too fat (my dad constantly berated me about my weight and once told me that I would grow up to be an alcoholic because I ate so much), just an "average" student, and not very popular—taken together, that was obviously why my father left. Why he stopped calling and coming to visit. Why I didn't see him for another twenty-five years.

Thanks to lots of therapy and maturity, I no longer play this game in terms of understanding why my father abandoned us . . . though I did have a bout of insecurity when, after making contact with my father decades later and meeting his "new" family, I saw that his two new daughters were thin.

I don't recommend playing the blame game, because it doesn't solve anything or help anyone. Unfortunately, however, the game can be compulsive, and though I always swear I'll stop playing, I keep going back to it.

Parents are notorious for playing. We play the blame game by connecting our parenting style to our child's behavior, the decisions our child makes (or doesn't make), and how our child ultimately "turns out."

As the mother of a child with neurodiverse and mental health challenges, I've played the game a lot and have met and heard from many others on this journey who do the same. In the "Special Needs/ Challenges Parents Edition" of the blame game, parents of children living with challenges blame themselves for their child's diagnosis, behavior, emotions, and actions. This game—some might call it a "match," a "bout," or a "scrimmage" or "tournament"—can never be won, but we play it anyway.

Playing the game puts parents in a kind of boxing ring with ourselves—only we are blindfolded and punching at an opponent we cannot see. We punch at decisions we made or didn't make that might have affected our child. We punch at incidents that happened that might have affected our child. We punch at the actions of other people that might have affected our child. We punch at circumstances that might have affected our child. We know this game will leave us bruised and bloodied, and yet we play it anyway.

Sometimes we play early in our journey, when we first get our child's diagnosis and it starts to sink in. Sometimes we don't have a diagnosis, but we suspect something and we start playing. Sometimes we completely forget about the blame game, but then something or someone reminds us that we haven't played in a while—maybe our child acts out, maybe someone asks us why our child behaves a certain way—and suddenly we find ourselves back in the ring.

Sometimes, we decide enough—we are not going to play anymore. But even when we make the decision to permanently step away from the game, there are these little nudges that can get us playing again.

Here are details of the blame game—the objective, rules, penalties, and accomplices/helpers involved in the game.

Objective of the Blame Game

What is the objective of the blame game? More importantly, why the hell do we even play it? Why would we use up so much of our precious time and energy on something that doesn't change the outcome? That doesn't change the challenges our child lives with?
The objective of the blame game, at least for me, is finding the "why." Ultimately, that's it—*why? Why* does my child live with these challenges, and what caused them? Surely there is a reason. After all, I am the mother, father, stepparent, grandmother, grandfather, auntie, uncle, or other caregiver, so the fault must lie with something I did or didn't do. Right?

You might think to yourself . . .
How could I have missed that?

If I had just . . . (here, you can fill in the blank with whatever mistakes you tell yourself you've made in your version of the blame game).

If I had only . . . (again, fill in the blank).

If this had happened or that hadn't happened, then things might be different.

Surely, I tell myself, if I can just answer all of these thoughts, then I will have achieved the objective of the blame game: finding the why.

Rules of the Blame Game

What are the rules of the blame game? Well, that depends on the person playing. For some, the rules are that everyone else is to blame. For others, a particular incident or circumstance is to blame. In my version of the blame game, my #1 rule is that all of the reasons for my daughter V's emotional and developmental challenges, all of the blame—it lies with me. All of the dots connect in a straight line pointing directly to me. It was something I did or didn't do, something I could have handled differently.

Penalities of the Blame Game

What are the penalties of the blame game? Perhaps the most significant is the crushing ton of guilt you are forced to carry. You blame yourself and constantly wonder:

What did I do?

What can I do to change this?
What did I miss?
Other penalties include: loss of sleep or sleeping too much, eating too much or not enough, isolating yourself, wearing yourself out taking care of others, and so on.

Helpers and Accomplices of the Blame Game

In the blame game, there are helpers and there are accomplices in the form of our friends, family, spouses, romantic partners, and coworkers. Sometimes even our own child (or children) can be either a helper or an accomplice.

Helpers don't want you to play the blame game. They see how damaging it is, and they don't want you to suffer or carry an undue burden. These people will see you playing and try to pull you out of the blame game. Helpers say things like:

"Don't blame yourself."
"Blaming yourself is only hurting yourself."
"Don't do that to yourself."

And then, on the other side of the field, there are the accomplices. These folks have no problem with you playing the blame game. In fact, they may get some kind of perverse satisfaction from watching you play. Accomplices may even push you further into the game by saying things like:

"Maybe it was your fault."
"Maybe if you had tried (insert unsolicited advice) . . ."
(See chapter 2 of this book.)
"Maybe you should have . . . (fill in the blank)."
"Maybe you shouldn't have . . ."

"You are the reason why . . ."

"If you had just . . . then (fill in another blank) wouldn't have happened." Beware of accomplices, because even though they may claim to mean well, they don't do anything to pull you out of the blame game. They only push you further in.

So, now that you know about the objectives, rules, penalties, and helpers and accomplices involved in the blame game, have you noticed there are no rewards to be gained from playing? That there is no way to actually win this game?

I'm going to use myself and my experiences as V's mother to show you how I play the game and—more importantly—how I always come up short, because as noted, the blame game cannot be won. Fortunately, I don't play as much as I used to, again thanks to therapy, supportive friends, and because as V has grown up, so have I. Over the years, I've realized that blame doesn't serve either of us—but sometimes I still want things to make sense in the way that $1 + 1 = 2$ does. And so, I play, because I struggle to understand that there are some things in life that will just never make sense—never. In my head, I know this to be true, but building a connection to my heart and making sure that connection flows freely hasn't quite happened yet. So, I continue to play and search, trying to figure out the why.

My version of the blame game involves a lot of "maybes":

Maybe it was the terrible blowout argument I had with my sister when I was around seven or eight months pregnant. I was so angry, so shaken up as a result. That could be why.

Maybe I should have stayed with the doctor I was seeing during the early part of my pregnancy with V (despite this doctor's cold, dismissive manner) instead of switching to a midwife whom I felt much more comfortable with and who had time for all of my questions. After all, a doctor would have induced before I hit forty weeks; the midwife waited too long. If we had induced, maybe the cord wouldn't have been wrapped twice around V's neck. She lost oxygen. That could be why.

Maybe I should have breastfed longer. I breastfed my oldest daughter, M, for fourteen months, but I ran out of steam after a couple of weeks with V and went to a combination of breastfeeding and formula, then all formula. Everybody knows breastfeeding is better, right? That could be why.

Maybe it was the divorce. I swore I wasn't going to put my children through a divorce, and I believed I had made the right choice in my partner so that wouldn't happen. So that my children would have two loving parents under one roof as I had not. So that they would have a father they weren't afraid of. While I accomplished that last part, as both my daughters aren't afraid of their father (actually, they have him wrapped round their fingers much of the time and feel safe with him), I still remember how V reacted after we told them that we were separating. V curled her eight-year-old frame into a corner of my home office and scratched out notes on yellow Post-its, then, one-by-one, walked over to my desk and handed them to me. One note read simply: "I didn't know." She didn't say a word to me then, just kept writing the notes and leaving them on my desk. That could be why.

Maybe it was the distant relative with all of the mental health stuff.

Maybe it was me. I have my own struggles with depression and anxiety.

Maybe it was something in my ex-husband's gene pool.

Maybe I . . .

Left her in front of the TV for too long.

Didn't read enough to her.

Should have fed her organic baby food instead of whatever baby food was on sale.

Was too distracted with my work.

Shouldn't have left her in that baby swing for so long while I cooked, cleaned, or just rested for a bit.

Didn't pay her enough attention.

Paid her too much attention

That could be why.

I've also dealt with not-so-good accomplices in my blame game. A friend who knew me well and witnessed the disintegration of my marriage once said to me:

"Do you think it was the divorce that caused all of this?"

I can't remember what my answer was, but I do remember that I was hella frustrated. Because how does a statement like that help? Was this person saying that after two and a half years of marriage counseling, my shattered marriage should be taped back together again? Was this person suggesting that we choke back all of the emotions that led to the admission that the marriage was over? That this act would have somehow changed V's diagnoses and behavior? Given her less challenges? In all my years of playing the blame game, I have never achieved the objective of the game. I have never figured out why V lives with these challenges, what caused them, or my role (or the role of others or particular circumstances) in them.

I have some theories, but they are just that—theories. I will never know the why, because I don't have a time machine that would take me back to the day V was conceived and allow me to do everything differently and then see what the results would be. None of us have time machines. None of us can go back and do it all over again. We can only move forward and love and support our children the best we can. I'm going to say that once again (maybe more for myself this time): *we can only move forward and love and support our children the best way we can.*

Before I finish this chapter, I want to specifically address one group of caregivers, a group that I am a proud member of: mothers.

Moms, for some reason, we are really good at playing the blame game. Whether or not we have a child living with challenges, we throw ourselves under the bus all the time. Maybe that's because we live in a world that seems to blame the mother for everything. We are the easy, satisfying target, the ultimate scapegoat.

"Did you see how well that young woman is doing? That's because of her mom. Good home training, that is."

"Did you read about what that kid did? That horrible thing that happened? I blame the mom; she had no control over him. She spoiled him. It's her fault."

Sometimes, when mind-bending incidents and situations happen involving our children, all eyes are on us.

And so I say this to my fellow moms out there: Let's do our best not to make any more contributions to the "Big Book of Blame" often assigned to us. I'm not saying we're perfect; I'm not saying we don't make mistakes, because like every other human being, we do. But let's try not to add to our personal blame book.

Now, you may be thinking, "Easier said than done," and I agree! However, I'm going to at least try.

Moms: I sit in support groups with you. I read about you. I see what you do to yourself and say to yourself, because I do and say similar things to myself. But maybe we can give ourselves a break. I'm not saying that we're going to completely stop blaming ourselves, but maybe we can just take a vacation from the blame game. And if we work hard at it, tell ourselves to stop when we notice it happening, and say to ourselves, "Playing the game isn't solving anything," then maybe, eventually, we can retire from it altogether.

Chapter 5 Takeaways

- Regardless of where we are on our journey of parenting a child living with challenges, we often blame ourselves for our child's struggles.

- Attempting to find the actual reasons for our child's challenges and diagnoses can prove impossible and only leads to further frustration and pain.

- Moms are especially good at playing the blame game, but in acknowledging this, they can also show themselves grace by reminding themselves that playing the game doesn't solve anything and won't help anyone.

For Further Thought

1. In what ways have you played the blame game in your life?

2. How has playing the blame game affected you?

3. In what ways can you free yourself from playing the blame game?

Self-Care Workshop – Play the Three Wishes Game

Make three wishes. Don't worry about time, expense, or feasibility—just think of three things that you wish for. The two rules of this game are: 1) each of your wishes *must* only focus on you (not your children, spouse, friends, parents, etc.), and 2) you can't wish for more wishes. Take a trip with your imagination and let your mind run free.

Chapter 6

The Forgotten Child

The Unique Challenges of the Siblings of Children Living with Mental Health and Neurodiverse Challenges

---

"In moving heaven and earth for one child, the sibling(s) of that child may feel overlooked and forgotten."

I was attending a support group for parents and caregivers of children with mental health and neurodiverse challenges when I first heard the term "forgotten child." I'd just finished sharing about the difficulties and frustrations I felt in balancing the needs of both of my children and feeling that my oldest daughter, M, often came up short in terms of the love, support, and attention she received from me and my former husband because we were so focused on her sister V's needs. The group leader referred to M as the "forgotten child," explaining that this is the term used when referring to the siblings of minor and adult children living with emotional, behavioral, developmental, and intellectual challenges.

I don't like calling M my forgotten child, as I think the term diminishes my love for her and how important she is to me and her father. However, I can't ignore the additional burdens placed on M as the result of being V's sister, because so much of M's life has been shaped by situations, decisions, and experiences involving V.

I'm going to tell you about an incident that happened between me and M that reminded me she is, indeed, my forgotten child, even if I cringe at the terminology.

First, a little background: I have severely arthritic knees. My right knee is bone-on-bone—that is, the cartilage is completely worn down, and my left knee isn't much better. On very bad days, I use a cane, and I even have one of those rectangular blue placards hanging from the rearview mirror of my car that allows me to park in spots for the disabled. I haven't come to terms yet with having that sign (or the cane), but I do love being able to avoid parking a football field away from the front doors of Costco.

Over the years, I've seen doctors about my knees and had the necessary interventions—anti-inflammatory pills, cortisone shots, gel injections, physical therapy—but the bottom line is that ultimately, I'll need to have both knees replaced. I hope to start the knee replacement process soon, but for now, I am forced to find whatever ways I can to ease the pain.

One way I found pain relief was a complete fluke. A friend of mine who knows of my never-ending battle with insomnia offered me some edible cannabis in chocolate form—a beautifully wrapped, expensive-looking candy bar you might give as a gift—because she said it helped her sleep. I was thrilled to try it to see if I might have similar results.

Unfortunately, the "dose" I took—a single square of chocolate that I broke off from the bar—did not make me sleepy, although I did find the most mundane things hilarious. I did notice, however, that after taking the edible, my knee pain practically disappeared. Wow—now that was a miracle!

Given my achy arthritic knees, you can probably guess that being on my feet for long periods of time leaves me in agony. Nonetheless, my kitchen looked as if a bomb had gone off in it, and since no one in my household seemed inclined to lift a finger to do anything about it, I decided to do a deep clean. Now, I mean the kind of deep clean that involves sponging down the inside (and outside) of the refrigerator, scrubbing the dried spaghetti sauce from inside the microwave, and matching the bottoms of the plastic storage containers with the tops.

The whole thing took me around three hours to complete, and when I was done, my knees were on fire. I decided to take more of the edible cannabis my friend gave me, but this time I doubled the dose and ate two squares plus a sliver more of the chocolate bar because I was really hurting. Knowing that relief was on the way, I limped through sweeping the living and dining rooms and then went up to my bedroom to sit down and answer some emails that had piled up.

The next thing I knew, I was having the worst anxiety attack I had felt in years. I was lightheaded, my heart was pounding, my mind was racing, and it seemed as if the bedroom was shrinking around me. And let me tell you, folks, I grew up with panic attacks before there was medicinal help for them, so I know what naked anxiety feels like, and this was bad.

V was at school and M, who was home doing college online due to the pandemic, knocked on my door and asked to come in. We'd been getting on each other's nerves lately and she wanted to come into my room to talk since we'd butted heads earlier that morning.

When M came in, I told her I was having a horrible anxiety attack and that I had taken double the amount of an edible to ease my knee pain. (No, I didn't hide the part about using an edible.) My daughter looked me over and said, "Mom, you took too much. You're high," which she found mildly amusing.

Trying to help me out, she Googled "antidotes for edible highs" (or something along those lines) on her laptop and brought me ice cubes for the back of my neck and pepper to sniff, because apparently ice cubes and pepper are supposed to cure a weed high. Neither worked. M then went downstairs and waited for V's bus to drop her off at our house. She told V some excuse—God knows what—and took her out for a few hours. When they returned, I was more myself. Still high, but able to fake the role of a mother who has herself together.

Now, the point of this story is not my aching knees or my inability to safely self-medicate. The point is the overwhelm and dread I saw in M's eyes as she watched me in my edible high—eyes that had seen and lost too much in her twenty years of living. It's about what I saw in her eyes as she watched me go from agitation to hysterical laughter to crying over incidents that happened in my childhood to frantically telling her over and over again that she had to make sure that V, who would be home from school soon, didn't see me like this. I told M that I needed her to cover for me—to meet V at the bus and keep her away from the house until I was back to myself again.

As V's sister, M has long been the Robin to my Batman (or Batwoman, in my case). She's been my reliable sidekick, my "go-to" whom I could count on to deal with whatever life threw at us. To absorb the emotional and sometimes physical blows of the journey of living with a sister with mental health and neurodivergent challenges. And I am well aware that this role—a role that she should not have had to play, but did so nonetheless—is a whole lot to put on a child.

It was M who covered for me while I became more myself as the effects of the edible lifted. But really, it's so much more than that. Because it was also M who, as a young child, would reluctantly step aside every time V would scream at her, bite her, or take a swipe at her when M wanted to do something as ordinary as hug me or feel love from me because V had (and has) an airtight attachment to me, unlike what would be considered typical between a mother and child.

As a result of V's inability to share me, M suffered the consequences. M instinctively knew that when V was near, the only way to keep the peace at home or in public was not to reach out to me for the hug she so desperately needed, not to hold my hand when the three of us walked together, not to say a simple "I love you, Mommy" if V was within earshot.

And truthfully, I didn't do much to address M pulling back because I wanted peace as well. You see, if V saw me show any kind of affection toward M, she would throw a tantrum that could only be compared to a Tasmanian devil on steroids. It felt like hours before we could get back to anything remotely close to "normal" after one of V's blowups.

So, as much as I dislike the phrase "forgotten child," I have to admit that from the early years of her life and even now, M has taken on that role.

So, what happens when a child learns to adapt to her sibling's behavior, even when that adaptation is unhealthy? Well, even now, twenty-plus years into this journey, when M and I embrace, I feel her start to pull away from me when V enters the room. It's become so natural now that I don't think M is even aware she does it.

In these moments, I purposely hold M longer and tighter just to show her that she matters and that she is loved. I can do this now because with therapy, medication, and time, V has made tremendous progress and is much better at accepting the loving bond I share with M. V still makes a stink about me showing M affection, but it's much more manageable.

Yet, so much damage has already been done. At times I feel helpless to do anything about it, because I was there. I was (and still am) a witness and a participant to the adjustments and modifications M makes in order to exist as V's sister. For years, I backed away from showing love to M when V started to blow. I would find M later, after V was taking a nap or out of the room, and I would see the swelling of small cuts on M's arms and know that those cuts were from when V dug her nails into M's flesh because M was trying to hug me. And I would hold M then, tell her how much I loved her, but the wounds—both physical and mental—were already made. The hurt was already there.

In the early years of this journey when V was in elementary school, she had major difficulty separating from me in order to go into the school building and comfortably settle into her classroom. And amongst all the hysteria that was a part of a typical school day morning (including what happened before we even got to school), M was there. M witnessed the bribing, cajoling, downright begging, frustration, and blowups (sometimes mine) that were a part of our daily routine to get V out the door and to school.

Some of V's loudest crying came when we tried to get her in the door of her classroom; she didn't want to let go of me. Each morning, within clear sight and sound of V's screaming and tears, was M's fifth grade class all lined up in single file, walking behind their teacher as she led them past V's classroom to the stairwell that led to their second-floor homeroom.

Remember those eyes filled with overwhelm and dread that I saw in M in the middle of my edible nightmare? I saw those same eyes every morning during elementary school. Every day, M's eyes were full of embarrassment and humiliation as she and her class marched past V in mid-tantrum. In these moments, I saw how M would try to shrink herself, almost make herself disappear when she walked by.

And sometimes, as M's teacher led the class to their classroom, the teacher would stop and ask V if she wanted to join the line with her older sister and sit with her in class for a few minutes so she could calm down. This was a loving, helpful gesture from M's teacher that worked. (I later learned that this teacher had a child of her own living with developmental challenges, so I can understand why she reached out in this way. She was on a similar journey herself.)

I don't know if it was the distraction of being with older kids or what, but V would go off with M to her classroom and eventually settle down. I welcomed this approach because although the school social worker and I had come up with a much better plan for me to hand off V in the mornings, at the time all I felt was relief that I could extricate myself from V and head out the door.

But guess who was left holding the reins?

I could go on and on with many more stories of incidents that happened throughout M's life and continue to this day to try and explain why M will always be my "forgotten child," but we would be here a long time.

All of this is why M's eyes haunt me. Because I know that somewhere in the mix of moving heaven and earth to help V, M got lost. And as I've already said, I also know that I was and still am an accomplice of sorts; I just wanted peace, and sometimes when I saw the yearning in M's eyes, I looked the other way.

M has always borne the weight of her sister's challenges and my trying to meet those challenges. This is not to say, of course, that her father and I don't love and cherish M and even spoil her. While I can't speak for my ex, I know that the spoiling I do is to make up for what she missed out on in her life and the guilt I feel about that.

I am a strong believer in therapy and made sure that M had a professional to talk to from a young age, and that continues to this day. I also keep the lines of communication between M and me wide open, and I often talk with her about how being in the role of a forgotten child affects her life and experiences as an adult. As painful as it can be for me as her mother, I acknowledge and receive the resentment M sometimes feels toward me and my parental role in her life. I think as parents, one of the best things we can do for our forgotten children is to honor their experiences and hold space for them to express what life was and is like for them.

And I'll also say this: Sometimes, I feel anger and resentment toward M, because I have worked my ass off to try and provide balance to a seesaw that has been tilted away from her. Sometimes I want to say: "Don't look at me like that. Don't get so angry at me. Don't you see how hard I'm trying (and have tried)?! Aren't I always available to talk about your feelings? About what makes you frustrated and angry? About what makes you happy? About what brings you joy?" Sometimes, I'll toss out evidence of my positive parenting:

"Didn't I start that Girl Scout troop from kindergarten and keep it together for years just so you could have the experiences of scouting? Heck, I don't even like camping, and if I see one more Girl Scout cookie I'll scream!"

"Haven't I always been your biggest cheerleader?"

But you know what? It doesn't matter, because this is about M's perceptions and lived experiences, not mine. So, when I see her eyes and I know what's clouded them, all I can do is take a deep breath, put my ego aside, and listen to her, be there for her and love her.

I asked M to read this chapter because I wanted to make sure that I accurately represented her feelings and experiences of being the sibling of a child living with emotional and developmental challenges. What she told me when she finished reading broke my heart because of the truth she spoke. She told me that when she hugs other people—not just me—that she pulls back from them because she feels there is a time limit, a love limit. She tells me that taking a back seat to V makes her feel like she doesn't have a story of her own because so much of her story is tied up with V's. M tells me that she feels responsible for V and worries about what will happen when me and my ex-husband are no longer alive. Will she have to take over caring for V?

I hem and haw when she says this, trying to think of an answer that will comfort her. I say that her dad and I have things set up so V will be cared for when we are gone, but I know those words don't resonate with M. I can see the fear in her eyes, the concern that she will never have a life of her own.

All I can do in this moment is listen to and love her.

I have spent countless hours talking to other parents and caregivers of children living with challenges who have similar experiences with their "forgotten children," who are in the constant struggle to provide balance for all of their children. What I've learned from these conversations is how common it is for siblings to feel "invisible" within the family dynamic and how important it is to honor and acknowledge those feelings and make room to discuss them, especially as the sibling grows and moves into and through adulthood.

As parents, it's not easy to balance loving and caring for all of our children, but we do the best we can under what feels like impossible circumstances.

Chapter 6 Takeaways

- Siblings of children living with mental health and neurodivergent challenges sometimes feel "invisible" or "forgotten" by their parents because of the amount of time and energy devoted to the needs of their sister or brother.

- Parents may feel overwhelmed with trying to see to the needs of all of their children and experience guilt that the neurotypical child was "left behind."

- The feelings and experiences of forgotten children must be acknowledged and honored.

For Further Thought

1. As parents, how do we live with and acknowledge the experiences of our "forgotten children"?

2. How do you think the experiences of being a forgotten child play out in adulthood?

3. How do you relate to the term "forgotten child"? What are your positive/negative feelings about it?

Self-Care Workshop – Take a Daily Vacation

Part of self-care is finding daily activities that give us a "vacation" from our everyday reality. Think about those daily activities that feel like small ways to escape—it might be taking a shower or a bath, taking a short walk, or having your favorite snack. Each day, decide on the activity that will be your temporary escape.

Chapter 7

Medicated

The Issues and Biases of Psychiatric Medication

"We all bring a lifetime of experiences and views on psychiatric medication to the table when thinking about whether or not to medicate."

Medication—both over-the-counter and prescription medication—is a big part of our lives. For the most part, we don't give it much attention. Got a headache? Pop some Tylenol. Period cramps? Take a couple of Advil. Hobbling through your day with sore arthritic knees? An Aleve should give you eight straight hours of relief. No big deal, right?

What about prescription medication? That stubborn cough that won't clear up despite your best home remedies turns out to be bronchitis and your doctor prescribes a course of antibiotics. After a couple of days, you are no longer coughing up a lung, and overall you feel better. Again, no big deal.

Chronic illness may require that we take prescription medication for a lifetime. Without it, our overall health will be in jeopardy. But even in these cases, there isn't much shame in sharing with family, friends, or complete strangers that we take daily insulin for diabetes, a pill to control our blood pressure, or medication for an underactive thyroid. We don't expect a "clutching of pearls" reaction to taking these medications. We don't whisper when we talk about these meds being a regular part of our life.

Consider, however, the difference in reaction, tone, and internal/external acceptance when talking about medication to treat anything having to do with the brain. When discussing medication for brain-related illnesses such as depression, anxiety, or a crippling mood disorder, it's pretty safe to say that the relaxed tone and easy exchange of information would not be the same.

What is it about medications associated with treating mental illness and other neurological challenges to the brain that brings about a tidal shift in attitude? That turns an open, conversational exchange of information into a whispered, shame-filled, closed-off one? That causes a negative shift in our opinion of someone who takes the medication?

Certainly, the way mental illness is portrayed as a whole in the media (usually negatively, with the scariest and most sensationalized storylines) has something to do with it. Maybe our personal feelings about psychiatric medication are shaped by all of the anecdotal information we've heard about it rather than what we actually know about the role it plays in people's lives.

As parents and caregivers on this journey, we often confront internal and external biases when considering medicinal help for our children (or for ourselves) that come from our life experiences—sometimes our very early experiences.

My opinions about all medications were developed as a child. I was raised with the belief that the only medication worth taking was in vitamin form. And I don't mean those cute, colorful Flintstones vitamins shaped like Fred and Barney; my mother would have none of that artificially flavored and colored nonsense. I mean the brown miniature-football-sized vitamins—specifically vitamin C—that could only be found in the 1970s local health food store that my mother frequented. (I still remember the smell of incense burning when we entered and the friendly barefoot owner who looked as if she'd stepped right out of a hippie commune.)

I had great difficulty swallowing pills, so my mother would crush up the vitamin C with freshly juiced apples and give the chalky, chunky, slightly sour mixture to me in a shot glass that I stared at for about an hour before summoning the courage to choke it back. It was disgusting.

To my knowledge, other than vitamin C and other vitamins named after letters of the alphabet, herbal remedies, and raw organic garlic—yes, garlic, which my mother believes cures everything—I don't know if my mom has ever taken an aspirin. I swear there is still a half-full bottle of Bayer somewhere in her home that has lived through seven presidents, and the only reason it exists is because either my sister or I snuck it into the house to help with menstrual cramps when we were teenagers. Medication for a young woman's monthly pain? Never! My mother believed that a good bowel movement, certain yoga poses, a heating pad, and, when necessary, a swig of brandy was better than any pharmaceutical aid.

If I had a cold, there would be no cold medication in our house. Instead, she rubbed Vicks VapoRub on my chest, neck, and with the tip of her index finger, placed a dab into each nostril, wrapped an old sock around my throat, and placed a hot water bottle on my chest. And, of course, she'd give me thousands and thousands of milligrams of vitamin C until the bug packed up and left my body.

Antibiotics? That doctor better have a damn good reason to prescribe them—like indisputable proof of a bacterial infection! And even then, she would prefer to go the herbal route.

To my mother's credit, according to a report from the Center for Disease Control (CDC), about one-third of antibiotic prescriptions are unnecessary. In fact, the overuse of these drugs has led to bacteria that have become resistant to this type of medicinal treatment. So, my mother's wisdom in terms of this particular prescription checks out.

In addition, it's hard to argue with my mother's logic in terms of medication, because she is very much alive and kicking. At ninety-one years old, she swims regularly, volunteers at her local food pantry, and looks at least twenty years younger. She is living proof of the value of natural remedies. (I will add, however, that she is genetically predisposed to longevity, as her father—my grandfather—lived until he was 103. Still, she embodies the argument against over-the-counter and prescribed medication.)

So, given my upbringing, medication felt taboo for much of my life. And as an extension of that, psychiatric medication made me break out in a cold sweat. Because if you're feeling depressed, my mother believes that taking a deep breath, sitting up straight, and doing meditation and yoga will cure it. No therapy and certainly no prescribed medication is needed.

When I was in my mid-twenties, a few years out of college and working at my first "real" job—in that it had a decent salary and came with health benefits and a retirement plan—the anxiety that had been a regular part of my life since I was nine became debilitating. Sinking into endless work projects, hours of exercise, and anything else to keep my mind busy no longer cut it. After working my day job, I was drained by the other job that required me to pretend I was okay when I was not.

So, despite feeling shame that I could no longer manage what was going on in my brain, I went to see a psychiatrist. (I had been seeing a psychotherapist, but she couldn't prescribe medication, which she thought I definitely needed.) The psychiatrist looked like a modern-day version of Sigmund Freud. I mean, he had the stern look, receding hairline, white beard, and round glasses—all of it. He asked me a series of questions while copiously scribbling notes onto a yellow legal pad. Based on the information I provided, he prescribed an anti-anxiety medication that I could take on an "as-needed" basis and warned me to use it sparingly because—and I'll never forget his words—"the brain thinks of this medication like it's candy," suggesting that the drug was highly addictive.

The doctor's words terrified me, but I was more terrified that I wouldn't be able to function and would lose my job (and the tiny New York City apartment that I was able to afford as a result of having said job). So, I took the prescribed medication.

The drug worked in that the anxiety I regularly felt was replaced by a relaxed, hazy feeling. The best way to describe it is that if someone had run into my office and excitedly told me that the building was on fire, I would have said, "Ok, thanks for letting me know," with a leisurely, unbothered tone and gotten back to work.

But I was so afraid of abusing the medication (and the possibility of becoming addicted) that I only used it when I was in extreme distress, and eventually I stopped taking it altogether. Back then, in the early 1990s, I wasn't aware of any type of "maintenance" medication that I could take daily to keep my anxiety at bay that would not become dangerously addictive. Certainly, those types of drugs were becoming more mainstream, but my fear that nothing could medically help me coupled with my inbred shame about taking psychiatric medication prevented me from doing the extra legwork to find out about it. So, I continued seeing my therapist and exercised like a madwoman, which helped keep the anxiety in check.

Then, in the early years of my daughter V's life—when I recognized that she was facing emotional and developmental challenges that I had not witnessed with my older daughter, coupled with the disintegration of my marriage—I found myself back in a psychiatrist's office in need of medicinal help for a brain that was not serving me very well. The weekly therapy sessions helped, but I needed more.

This time, I was prescribed a daily medication that seemed to be the "drug of the day" in that I had read about it in magazines and seen commercials on TV about it. I remember one commercial featured a downtrodden-looking woman dragging her weary frame through her daily activities (there's even a rain cloud over her head for effect) and then, after taking the medication, the cloud is replaced by the sun as the now joyous woman breathes in the sweet aroma of a bouquet of flowers and then plays fetch with a golden retriever. I wanted to be that woman, so I began taking the medication.

Instead of relaxed, sun-drenched days traipsing through flower beds with a dog trotting along at my heels, however, my experience on the drug made my anxiety worse and brought on a type of extreme paranoia that I had never experienced before. And that's the hard part

71

about medication—what works for one person may have an opposite, very different effect on another, and God knows why. Perhaps it's blood type? Genetics? Bad luck?

I called the doctor after a few days on the drug and told him that I felt as if I was losing my mind. My usual fears were amplified, and I had a looser grip on reality. The doctor, who hadn't been recommended to me but was on my insurance plan, told me that he had started me on a "Mickey Mouse" amount of the med (his words for a low dose) and told me that I "should not be having such a reaction." His lack of understanding and support made me feel worse, as if it was somehow my fault that the drug wasn't working. What an asshole.

At any rate, the doctor told me to stay on the medication and that the side effects would pass. But they didn't, and soon I stopped taking it and gave up (perhaps prematurely) on finding a pill what would help me. When I think back to that time, I realize that what I needed most was to find a psychiatrist who was patient with me as we worked together to find a medicinal solution to my mental health issues. Having that kind of connection is essential. I also needed to be a better advocate for myself and tell the doctor that we needed to try something else (despite being on a low dose), but I had found it difficult to self-advocate when I felt so psychologically unstable.

And so, I continued on playing the role of someone who felt happier than she actually was, which was exhausting.

Then, about two years later, I hit a wall of anxiety and depression that all of the weekly (sometimes twice weekly) therapy sessions and exercise in the world could not get me over. So, I went to a different psychiatrist, one who didn't take my insurance but came with a solid recommendation from a friend. This doctor listened attentively to my story, diagnosed me with clinical depression, and said that no one should have to live the way I had been living (that is, barely hanging on).

He told me that there were many psychiatric medications that I could try and that we just needed to find the right one. He advised me to be patient throughout the process of finding a good medicinal fit and also recommended that, if possible, I talk to a close blood relative, preferably a sibling or parent, who suffers with similar psychiatric issues as mine and find out what (if any) medication they took for it. If that med worked for them, it may just work for me. This particular recommendation was easier said than done, but I did get some family medicinal information and started on a low dose of the same medication. After tolerating the lower dose, I moved to a higher dose.

At first, I didn't recognize the effects, as some psychiatric medications need to build up in the system before any remarkable change can be felt. But eventually, I noticed that my emotional mountains weren't as steep. They were still there, but I felt I could more easily get over them. My mind raced less. My anxieties became more manageable. Things I had trouble doing because of anxiety—like driving on the highway and over bridges—became doable.

I felt less guilty, less responsible for the bad things that happened in my world—which was a small miracle since, in some way or another, I felt as if an invisible cord tied me to every misfortune in my life. In my mind, everything was my fault. Divorce? My fault. Struggling child? My fault. Family dysfunction? My fault. Work issues? My fault. A bit grandiose, I admit, but a true feeling that I was happy to lessen.

Perhaps the greatest affirmation I can give to being on medication is that if someone told me that I would have less time on this earth because of the medication I take (which has never been proven, but

I'm trying to make a point here), I would tell them that I would gladly forfeit those years to live with a peaceful brain.

So, given my journey with medication, you would think I would have no problem with my daughter needing psychiatric medication, right? Wrong. I felt shame. I felt like I had messed up as a parent. She was just a young child then, not even a teenager. My kid, on medication? I was already hearing all these scary possible diagnoses from doctors attempting to identify why she struggled so much.

Yes, I could take meds, but not my kid. What would the lasting effects be on her young body? Would it affect her physical development? Brain development? How long would she need to be on meds?

But all my fears about the medications and their effect on V could not match the level of emotional pain she was in. Her mind had become her enemy. Yes, we had her in therapy and involved in various activities, made adjustments to her diet, and tried every other non-medicinal intervention, but more had to be done.

So, our journey to finding the right combination and dosage of medications began—what parents and caregivers sometimes refer to as finding the right "cocktail" of medications. It can take quite some time to get this cocktail just right, and even then, adjustments often need to be made.

We tried a little bit of this and a little bit of that. We tried a lot of that and lowered some of this. Sometimes it was a lot of that in the morning, a bit of this in the afternoon, and then more of that at night. Sometimes this made her overly tired; sometimes that made her body twitch. Sometimes this and that together caused weight gain. Once, that caused my preteen daughter to lactate.

We tried the thin white round pills, the thick white round pills, the white oval pills, the thick white round pills with the thin white round pills. We tried half the oval pill with the thick white round pills. We added the blue round pills, then the green-and-yellow capsules.

The orange pills worked great for a while, but then they didn't. We tried the white round pill with the little blue pill. We increased the dose of the orange pill, which we balanced with the round disk-shaped white pill.

And then we were told we should try *that* medication. That medication? You want to put her on that? That medication we whisper about but don't say out loud? That old medication that's been around since the mid-twentieth century? That one that I heard about, always negatively, in the movies? You've got to be kidding me, right? If I were to use sound effects to convey the moral judgment I attached to this particular medication, you would now hear the brittle crack and deep boom of thunder.

But I trust and respect V's psychiatrist, who always listens patiently to my concerns, so . . . we tried that medication. And guess what? It worked. We had to make some adjustments with the dosage, but it worked! And when I say "it worked," I don't mean that V was suddenly and miraculously a different child who didn't suffer from emotional and developmental challenges. What I mean is that her mind became more of her friend. Her mind became more manageable and less draining to her. The hamster wheel thinking patterns of her brain slowed, and reasoning with her became easier. She could quiet her mind enough to sit in her room and read a book.

And I have to brag a bit—this particular parental brag is better suited to this chapter than other bragging forums (like Facebook). Unlike me, who had to have pills chopped up with apple juice so I could swig them back, with at least one or two gagging episodes as a kid, V is a master at swallowing pills. When she first went on her meds, her psychiatrist gave us a glossy blue index card with cartoon characters on it that explained different ways to swallow pills. One of the techniques—blowing up her cheeks with pills and a huge gulp of water and pretending to be a puffer fish—became her favorite.

Now, are we done with medication adjustments? No. Because that's not our reality. V's brain continues to grow and mature, and we will have to continue to work with this pill and that pill in various combinations for the rest of her life. Medications have to be adjusted and changed; that's a reality. I am grateful that we live in a time when these meds are readily available, and I can only hope that with continued research, even better medications will someday become available to V and the countless other people who live with illnesses and challenges that affect the brain.

Do I read the reams of paper that come with the bottles of pills about all the associated side effects? No. Hell no. Because if I did, I would be too scared to give her anything. Instead, I remove the medicine bottles from the white paper bag and toss the associated paperwork in the shredder. I don't worry about all of the horrible side effects, because we always start on a low dose, watch her like a hawk, and are prepared to make a change if something doesn't appear to be working. I go by how she acts and feels, not what's printed on those dreadful lists of side effects. I understand that side effects are a necessary evil with the medications V takes, but I also understand that the benefits far outweigh the risks.

With all the years of experience I have with psychiatric medication, you would think that I would be more vocal about it, not whisper or otherwise lower my voice when discussing it. That witnessing the positives and how they outweigh the negatives in my and V's life might even cause me to shout the names of the medications from my rooftop. But I don't.

I feel self-conscious when I forget to stow away V's seven-day pill organizer, accidentally leaving it on the bathroom counter in full view for guests to see all the pills placed in the AM and PM sections. On those occasions when I spend the night with a romantic partner and need to take my meds before bed, I duck into the bathroom instead of pulling them out in plain sight and risking an unwanted discussion of why I take them.

I could probably create some kind of avant-garde art sculpture with all of the empty amber-colored medicine vials I have never thrown away but instead stuff into plastic bags and put under beds and in the back of closets. Why not just toss the empty vials into the recycling bin like I do empty Tylenol, Advil, cough syrup, and antibiotic containers? Because it takes too much time to peel off the identifying Rx labels, and I have this fear that during one of the all-too-frequent windstorms that seem to pass through on recycling day, my blue storage bin will blow over with all of its contents scattered onto the lawns of my neighbors. As they dutifully clean up the accumulated mess—all of the empty tin cans, spaghetti sauce bottles, cardboard boxes, and old newspapers—everyone will see that we medicate.

We all bring a lifetime of experiences and views on psychiatric medication to the table when thinking about whether or not to medicate. Your decision to medicate or not medicate your child is just that—your decision. I made certain choices for myself and V that I stand by, because those choices have improved our lives. But whatever your decision is, that's your business, not mine. As always, just do the best you can.

Chapter 7 Takeaways

- A double standard exists in terms of medications used for chronic physical illnesses, such as diabetes, and medications that treat chronic issues related to the brain.
- Our opinions about psychiatric medication have a lot to do with our personal experiences.
- Finding the right combination of medications to treat brain-related illnesses takes time, and that combination may need to be adjusted over time.
- The ultimate decision on whether to medicate your child is deeply personal.

For Further Thought

1. How do you think your views about psychiatric medication have been shaped by your personal experiences and/or the opinions of others?

2. What thoughts come to mind when you think about psychiatric medication? How have those thoughts changed based on being on this journey with a child or loved one living with challenges?

3. Who in your life (friends, family, work colleagues, etc.) would you feel comfortable talking with about your child taking psychiatric medication? Why? Who would you not feel comfortable having this conversation with? Why?

Self-Care Workshop – Music Therapy

Most of us have a song or two that makes us feel good and uplifts our mood. Think of the tune(s) that makes you feel great and listen to it. Trust me, you'll be glad that you did!

Chapter 8

The Things We Celebrate

Acknowledging and Honoring Unique and Nontraditional Milestones of the Journey

---

"As parents and caregivers of minor and adult children living with challenges, our celebrations and special moments deserve to be acknowledged, honored, and observed, no matter how unusual or insignificant they may seem."

When my daughter V turned eighteen, we celebrated by going out to dinner at her favorite Japanese Hibachi restaurant, where a chef cooked our dinner tableside on a giant iron grill. To our collective "oohs" and "aahs," the chef performed a juggling act with spatulas, made a volcano choo choo train out of an onion, and demonstrated his expert knife skills while preparing our steak, chicken, and shrimp dinners. We all had a great time.

But that same day, there was a *different* celebration for me that I only shared with close friends of mine who knew of the bumpy journey that had brought V to this milestone birthday. What was this additional celebration?

That V was alive and had made it to eighteen years old.

That she'd made it despite the dangerous decisions and situations she had put herself in. Despite the multiple times she had threatened to kill herself. Despite the debilitating depression, anxiety, and delusions that had resulted in multiple visits to the emergency room and eventually landed her in a residential home for emotionally and behaviorally challenged children for nearly a year when she was just twelve years old.

V had made it to eighteen, and I celebrated because for so long, I had feared that this day would never come and lived with the darkness of that possibility.

Most of us celebrate holidays, graduations, birthdays, weddings, anniversaries, a new home or job, the birth of a child—it's expected. We mark these special occasions with formal parties, big and small get-togethers, a meal at a favorite restaurant, and, with what has become a tradition of the twenty-first century, posts on social media. In fact, you can pretty much tell the time of year by the celebratory posts and photos you see on Facebook, Instagram, TikTok, or whatever platforms you frequent.

Folks dressed in caps and gowns? It's graduation time, probably May or June. Freshly scrubbed kids in new clothes with backpacks slung over their shoulders and mini bottles of hand sanitizer hanging off the side? It's the first day of elementary school, usually August or September. A beautifully roasted turkey with all the trimmings and too many side dishes to count placed at the center of a large dining room table crowded with family and friends? It's Thanksgiving, the end of November.

Celebrations are a part of our lives, and like everyone else, parents and caregivers of children living with challenges have celebrations too. But some of those celebrations are not captured in a photograph and posted on social media. You won't see family and friends dressed in their finest clothes raising their glasses in a toast to the big accomplishment.

These celebrations—we might call them "special moments," "things we thought would never happen," or "things we hold on to but fear they might slip away"—are different from what we consider to be "mainstream" celebrations, but they are still important and worthy of recognition. These special moments are different because the significance and gravity of them don't fit into the celebrations most people are accustomed to and comfortable with.

I have lots of celebrations that you won't find a Hallmark card for. For example, I celebrate that V regularly takes her psychiatric medication because I know very well that medication compliance— that is, the willingness to regularly take medicine—is not a given on this path. Many parents and caregivers agonize over their minor or adult child's refusal to consistently take medication, even though that medication may settle a racing mind, lift a depressed spirit, or calm debilitating anxiety.

Can you imagine the social media post I could make to celebrate? Perhaps a photo of a smiling V holding a glass of water in one hand as she reaches toward the seven-day AM/PM medication organizer on the dining room table filled with all the multicolored and multishaped pills she takes. I'd put a bouquet of red and yellow roses next to the pill organizer, tie some pink balloons to a nearby chair, and post the following:

"Overwhelming week is gonna be a bit easier with the help of these assorted gems. My kid is a consistent pill-chugging rock star!"

I wonder what kind of reaction I would get to that celebratory post. I'd hope for at least a few "likes."

Or perhaps your child has what seems like an unbreakable attachment to a particular piece of clothing, but that piece of clothing needs to be washed or switched out for something more weather-appropriate. Finally—several meltdowns later, just before you've given up hope of ever replacing the clothing—your child puts on the new clothing and keeps it on. Hallelujah! Break open the bottle of champagne and start your happy dance!

Sometimes changes to our child's behavior are so subtle that we don't notice the shift in their demeanor or attitude right away. Reasoning with V is impossible at times because her mind and thinking patterns can be on a continuous loop. In this state, logic goes out the door: 2 + 2 = 9, night does not follow day, and there are seventeen months in a year. Our conversations, often heated, feel upside-down.

I've noticed, however, that with getting V's medication cocktail just right, along with intensive therapy and maturity, our conversations— even the confrontational ones—feel more manageable. Her mind still loops, but it's gotten much better. And for that, I celebrate. I remind myself of how far she and I have come on this path and pour a little more wine into my glass, buy myself a new book, or just sit and marvel at the wonders of my precious child. In fact, I just may celebrate with a social media post where I place side-by-side photos on Instagram—one of a tsunami wave standing thirty feet high, about to crash down on a city, and the other of a much smaller wave with a surfer riding it. The accompanying post could read:

"Happy to be surfing the waves with my sweet daughter, not crushed by them."

Would people respond to my post with hearts and thumbs-up emojis?

Here are some other special moments that those on this road might celebrate:

- A teenager lost in depression smiles, and for the briefest of moments her spirit is lighter. Whoo-hoo and thank God, because you had no idea this would happen given how bleak things have been for her.

- A child overwhelmed with anxiety makes it through an entire school day. Absolutely *no* calls from the school nurse telling you to come pick up your child and bring him home. Cue the applause!

- A mother applying for services for her son completes and sends in countless forms, only to receive a note from a government agency that she needs to send in more forms, only to be told that the original forms she sent were lost and she needs to send them again, only to hear that the services she is applying for are denied. But she takes a deep breath, has a good cry, punches some pillows, and then reapplies. And the second time (or perhaps the third), the services she so desperately needs to support her child are approved. Time for a party and a victory lap around the corner!

- Perhaps *absolutely nothing* has happened in a single day—no verbal explosions or meltdowns, no threats, no walls punched in. Just an ordinary day. For that, we celebrate.

On this journey, our celebrations are often tinged with caution, because what we celebrate feels fragile. We wonder how long it will last. We may tiptoe through these special times and knock on wood in the hopes that the behavioral changes will stick. We may not utter words of gratefulness or breathe a sigh of relief for fear of jinxing what we see before us. We may feel that somehow, acknowledgement of any kind will take away what we so desperately hope for.

Sometimes family and friends who are not on this journey have no clue as to why we celebrate. They wonder how we could rejoice in a particular event that seems ordinary to them or may even appear to warrant more grief than celebration. But we know why—although we may be too overwhelmed and exhausted to connect to the enormity of the smallest of changes.

A close friend of mine on this journey had a particular celebration that was shadowed with caution, but it was a celebration nonetheless. Her daughter, who lives with emotional and behavioral challenges, has spent much of the past few years in residential treatment programs, but for the past several months she has lived at home with her mother and younger sister. Despite all that was put in place to support this major transition—a psychiatric team, including a case manager and in-home therapist, a therapeutic school that includes even more psychiatric support, and medication—her daughter will not stay home.

She'll say she's leaving for a couple of hours and instead is gone for several days, sometimes weeks. Where she goes and who she's with is mostly a mystery, but it's almost always with someone she meets on the Internet who offers to pick her up, send an Uber to an agreed upon spot, or send her money for transportation. In the rare times that her daughter is home, she is verbally abusive to her mother and sister, refuses to attend school with any consistency, and does not regularly take her medication.

Needless to say, my friend has been emotionally devastated by the struggles of her daughter—the disappearances and then reappearances, sometimes at my friend's doorstep, sometimes at a local police station, sometimes on the side of a road many miles (or states) away. When her daughter returns, she has often been mentally, physically, and sometimes sexually abused. And it is my friend who takes her to the hospital for evaluation and, along with a psychiatric team, tries to convince her not to leave home. But it's as if her daughter hears a siren's song calling to her, and she follows it and leaves home again.

Most recently, when her daughter returned home from being away for several days, my friend placed her in a residential facility again. But because she turned eighteen while in the facility, this young woman had the legal right to check herself out, which she did. And, as expected, she disappeared again.

This time when her daughter reached out to her from the road for help, my friend told her that she's welcome to come home if she gets regular psychiatric treatment, attends high school, takes her prescribed medication, and follows the rules of the household. If she could not do this, then she could not come home. Upon hearing this, my friend's daughter hurled a litany of expletives at her mother and physically threatened her. But my friend knows that however heart-wrenching it is to set these rules and boundaries, it is the only way to help her daughter.

When I met with my friend for coffee and to catch each other up on what was going on in our lives, I was pretty sure that she would tell me her daughter was gone again, because this has been the pattern.

But here's the celebration part of this story: Much to her and my surprise, my friend told me that her daughter contacted her and said she is checking into a homeless shelter for people ages eighteen to twenty-one in our area. For the moment, at least, she was no longer on the run. My friend's daughter had said she wanted to make changes in her life, make better choices.

Someone not familiar with the heartbreak, agony, and dashed hopes of having a child with psychiatric challenges who frequently disappears may not recognize the significance of my friend's daughter checking herself into a homeless shelter and wanting to make a change, but we do.

What will happen next? We don't know. Will she run again? We don't know. But for now, we give thanks and, however shakily, celebrate this moment over coffee and tears.

So, celebrate that your child made it to school. Celebrate that your trip outside the home with your child went smoothly without any meltdowns. Celebrate that your child who has struggled with sleep is now sleeping, so now you can sleep. Celebrate that you were able to take a walk and breathe. Celebrate that you let go of negative feedback from others that has weighed you down. Celebrate that you cried, and in those tears, you felt the relief of letting go and accepting that you are only human.

As parents and caregivers of minor and adult children living with challenges, our celebrations and special moments deserve to be acknowledged, honored, and observed, no matter how unusual or insignificant they may seem.

Chapter 8 Takeaways

- What we celebrate as parents and caregivers of children living with challenges is often very different compared to more traditional celebrations.

- Nevertheless, it is important that we recognize and honor even the smallest (and what may feel like unique or unusual) victories on this path.

For Further Thought

1. As a parent or caregiver, what have you celebrated that is different from what might be considered a "traditional" celebration? How did you celebrate?

2. In what ways can you celebrate yourself as a parent or caregiver on this journey?

3. What new celebratory traditions would you like to see in your life?

Self-Care Workshop – Celebrate You

When was the last time you gave yourself a compliment or honored your accomplishments? Congratulate yourself for something you accomplished today! Did you get enough sleep (or take a much-needed nap), drink plenty of water, or enjoy a cup of tea? All of these activities are worthy of celebration because you took care of you.

Chapter 9

Punching Bag

When Parents Become Emotional Punching Bags

"It is common to feel like an emotional punching bag on the journey of loving and advocating for a child living with challenges."

In this journey as parents and caregivers, we may feel like lightning rods that attract criticism, blame, and judgment from those closest to us or even total strangers. I recently saw a video of young boy, maybe around twelve or thirteen, running onto a football field in the middle of an NFL game. Needless to say, this was a big deal, as it disrupted the game. Security quickly grabbed the child (more like pummeled him) and escorted him off the field.

Sporting events are sometimes interrupted by protesters looking to make a statement, electrified fans, or even stray animals. It's a spectacle, for sure, but not completely unexpected. However, what struck me about this particular incident was a comment posted by a sportscaster covering the game that read:

"What kind of parent lets their kid run onto the field?"

Now, I don't know the specifics of the story and all that was involved, but I highly doubt the child's parent (or whomever he was with) pointed him toward the field crowded with players, coaches, officials, and press and yelled:

"Ready, set, go!"

Yet, without knowing the backstory, this commentator decided that the parents were to blame. And unfortunately, it is extremely common for parents and caregivers to take the emotional blows for their child's reactions, moods, and struggles.

Imagine a child has a meltdown in a supermarket, restaurant, or other public place. While the parent frantically tries to soothe her child and get some control over the situation, she can't ignore the stares, glares, and nasty whispered comments, such as:

"She needs to control her child."

Imagine an older child frequently has run-ins with the law, struggles with addiction, or continually makes choices that land them in trouble. Quite often, there is an invisible finger pointing at the parent. The blame and accusations come from outsiders (and sometimes from those within our orbit) who don't understand the sharp twists, turns, and overall bumpiness of the road that is mental illness and addiction. It's as if we as parents and caregivers are mere punching bags—objects for people to take aim at and release their judgment, misunderstanding, and rage.

Now, you probably know what a punching bag is, but just in case you don't, here are the two definitions from Merriam-Webster:

1. A stuffed or inflated bag usually suspended for free movement and punched for exercise or for training in boxing.
2. One who is routinely abused or defeated by another.

When I use the term "punching bag" here, I mean a version of the second definition.

Of course, being a punching bag is not reserved solely for parents and caregivers of children living with challenges. At times, almost everyone feels like a punching bag in one way or another—unfairly blamed, scapegoated, attacked, or misunderstood. Perhaps it was a work situation or something that took place in school, within a circle of friends, with a family member, or with a romantic partner. In those times we may feel humiliated, disrespected, unappreciated, unheard, and unloved.

We can—hopefully—try to do something about it. We can confront or distance ourselves from the person and/or situation. Maybe we accept the situation, as hard as it is, knowing that it will eventually end. Maybe we leave the job, end the abusive relationship, or find a new friend.

But sometimes, it seems there is no end to being an emotional punching bag. That the dynamic just becomes a regular part of our lives, has a chair at our dinner table, and walks alongside us wherever we go.

This is a reality faced by many parents and caregivers of children living with challenges. And as a result, we feel worn down and worn out.

Sometimes the punches come not from an outsider, but from our own child, either intentionally or unintentionally. Like when, for instance, conversations and disagreements stay on a continuous loop in which reality takes a back seat to delusions and paranoia. When boundaries necessary for all involved are continuously crossed. When promises are broken and offers of help ignored. When our beloved child says or does things that hit us in the most sensitive places of our heart.

I often feel like an emotional punching bag when it comes to the relationship with my youngest daughter, V. Why do I feel this way? Well, there's lots of "whys," but the main one is that she often sees me as her enemy and feels my actions are somehow against her when I am her greatest advocate.

For the life of me, I just can't understand why parents—mothers in particular—get hit the hardest and the most. Why is the person who is on the frontlines advocating for and loving a child most often the recipient of the blows?

In support groups and from other parents on this path, I hear that it is because we are our child's "safe" place. We are the person who will not abandon them, who will always be there for them, and therefore our child feels they can take out their pain, frustration, and aggression on us. I get it, but it doesn't make me feel any better. The cumulative effects of being V's punching bag leaves me feeling like I've actually gone a few rounds in the ring with the most skilled of boxers.

And I also understand that V's behavior is the result of her having an illness that affects her brain, but still, that doesn't give me much relief. It doesn't help me feel any less beaten up.

And when life is good between me and V—that is, when our day-to-day life as mother and daughter is stable (or as stable as it can be under the circumstances)—I feel like I am sitting on a rickety chair that will collapse at any moment under the weight of whatever emotional rollercoaster comes next.

Maybe your child *doesn't* think of you as the enemy, but you are in a daily battle to get them to admit they need help, regularly take their medications, see a therapist, or enter a rehabilitation program. Perhaps you are punch-drunk from listening to continuous cycles of profanity-laced outbursts followed by apologies and then more attacks.

Maybe you've had so many blows that hope—the hope for change, hope for peace, hope for the future—gets knocked out of you.

I've become close with another mom on this path whom I met a few years ago at a support group. We regularly get together for coffee to trade battle stories about our children, rejoice in the smallest of victories, and have whooping belly laughs over our attempts at online dating. My friend sometimes talks about the difficulty she has with maintaining hope that things will change for her daughter. About the cycle of being an emotional punching bag for her child. In her words, "hope hurts."

Hope seems so simple, right? We just have to have hope—to believe in positive outcomes, to trust in better days no matter how many blows we've sustained on this journey. Never give up hope, hold on—it's a mantra heard all the time, from friends, family, doctors, therapists, religious leaders, neighbors, and even strangers. It seems as if almost every affirmation on social media starts with hope. Yet what happens when that hope has been beaten to a pulp? When having hope brings more pain than relief? When hope feels like a sucker punch straight to the gut?

Parents aren't supposed to lose hope in their children. Although you may sometimes hear parents jokingly say, "I give up," that's a no-no in the big book of parenting.

But what if, after years of being on an emotional and sometimes physical battlefield with a child, the statement "I give up" feels real rather than just some throwaway words said in frustration? When feelings of hopelessness morph into acceptance of our realities, because that's all we can do?

We can try to remember that it is the illness and its effects that are striking us, not our child. Lately, however, that hasn't been working for me, but I keep it in my back pocket and try to remember it.

Something that I find helpful is to keep a continuous gauge on myself and where I am in terms of getting enough sleep, eating well, and taking time to do something that I enjoy, like reading, watching a favorite program, or listening to music that heals me. I acknowledge that when my tank is empty and when I have not been taking good care of myself, that is when I feel the effects of being V's punching bag the most. It is then that my interactions with V are the most counterproductive—like staying with her in looping, never-ending arguments instead of walking away, or losing my temper and saying something I know I will regret later.

I'm not saying that it ever feels good to be a punching bag for V's emotions, but I can sure ride the waves better when my tank has some gas in it. I can see the blows coming and change the subject, divert the conversation to another topic. Take a deep breath and gently say, "Ok, I hear you," or, "Let's talk when I'm in a better mindset," instead of losing my composure and going down the rabbit hole of an argument with her.

It also helps to remind myself that I am not that person she is accusing me of being; I am not "evil" (one of V's favorite accusations). It helps to speak with trusted friends who know me well and who remind me that I am doing the best I can. Who remind me not to believe the vitriol that is being spit out at me.

Sometimes it helps me to look at photos of V when I'm away from her. The photographs, taken at different stages of her life, help to remind me of the boundless love I feel for her. They remind me of her many accomplishments. They remind me of how far she and I have come on this journey. Looking at them gives me my daughter. It lets me spend time with her alone, without judgment—hers or mine—and appreciate this person whom I helped bring into this world.

Sometimes, we—not our children—can even be our own punching bags. We punch ourselves for losing our temper, for feeling deep resentment toward our child, for wanting to run away from it all, for imagining a different life. We punch ourselves for having feelings toward our child that are counterintuitive to what it means to be a parent.

And when these inevitable feelings arise, I'll say to you what I often say to myself: *Give. Yourself. A break.* You are human, and these feelings—feelings that someone not on this path may have trouble understanding—are to be expected. When they come, don't beat yourself up over them. Try to understand and accept that they are part of this bumpy journey and that you are only human.

Most of us on this path feel like punching bags at times. But it is my hope that you can find ways to feel like less of a punching bag or get an entire reprieve from the feeling. No matter what your journey entails, just know that I'm right there with you.

Chapter 9 Takeaways

- Parents of children living with challenges may feel as if they are their child's personal punching bag, which can lead to emotional numbness and exhaustion.

- Sometimes parents can be their own worst punching bag.

For Further Thought

1. In those times when you have felt like a human punching bag, how did you react? Would you change any of the ways you reacted? If so, how and why?

2. When you have been your own punching bag—when you've given yourself an especially hard time over something that happened in your life—how could you have been easier on yourself?

3. What words of comfort would you say to a dear friend who feels like a punching bag? Can you imagine saying those same words to yourself?

Self-Care Workshop – Try "Skychology"

Skychology is the act of gazing up at the expansiveness of the sky and using that feeling of wonder to enhance our overall well-being. In our day-to-day lives, we may sometimes feel closed in or trapped by our reality and our circumstances. A momentary release from this feeling is to go to the nearest window or, if possible, go outside and simply look up at the vastness of the sky. Notice the blueness, the grayness, the cloudiness, the light or the darkness, and its wide expanse. Doing so can help us "zoom out" and see ourselves and our emotions within a much larger context, which can bring about more positive feelings.

Chapter 10

Surviving and Thriving

Living Fully While on the Journey

"There is a place somewhere between surviving and thriving where parents and caregivers of minor and adult children living with challenges can live, breathe, and grow."

How has your life been this past week? Would you say you survived? Thrived? Or somewhere in the middle? To survive (according to the Merriam-Webster dictionary) is to live and exist within our day-to-day lives, despite the inevitable hardships and challenges we may face. Compare that definition to the one for thriving: to prosper; to grow, develop, and flourish as human beings; to meet goals we have set for ourselves and grow personally and spiritually; to feel peaceful and contented. So, are you surviving or thriving?

This week, I bounced back and forth between surviving and thriving, although I've definitely spent many years in solid survival mode. For me, the sweet (and realistic) spot is somewhere in between, but definitely leaning more toward thriving. Let's call this place "surthrival."

Parents and caregivers of minor and adult children living with challenges certainly know what it is to survive while living alongside daily, significant, and sometimes debilitating struggles and challenges. We do it every day on this journey. We continue to put one foot in front of the other and push on. We navigate through the meltdowns, crises, and uncertainty, doing the best we can.

Is it possible, however, to do *more* than just survive on this path? To do more than just keep our heads above water and not go under? I often pose this question to friends of mine on this journey and to myself. That is, are we destined to just survive—to simply hold on for dear life and put out fires—or can we actually thrive? Can our lives have some meaning outside of the overwhelm and exhaustion of our realities? Can we follow our dreams, achieve our personal goals? What does that look like? What does that feel like?

I consider myself to be a late bloomer in life. High school, college, and much of my adult life were not my shining hours; I don't look back at these times with particularly fond memories. I experienced the ups and downs of life like everyone else. There were still accomplishments and major life-changing events, but for much of this time, I felt disconnected from myself. I existed in a world with a strict, self-imposed playbook of rules and regulations on how to be the best mother, wife, daughter, sister, friend, girlfriend, lover, neighbor, and worker. This playbook was not focused on my own needs and happiness, but instead focused on and gave significant weight to how good I made others feel. If the other people in my life were good—if I catered to their needs and ignored my own, or perhaps pretended that their needs were my needs—then all was good in my world. It was a suffocating existence, but one I lived within and which I became all too comfortable with.

I finally bloomed, so to speak, in my fifties. By "bloomed," I mean that after years of therapy (and discovering some very good anti-depressants), I was able to come to terms with painful parts of my early life and understand how those experiences influenced the choices I made, how I lived my life, and the extent to which I gave other people power to decide my own happiness and well-being. I was finally able to loosen my grip on that unforgiving playbook that put others' needs before my own. As a result, significant relationships in my life changed, and some ended—and that was and is a price that I willingly pay for the peace I now feel. I am less fearful of life, more trusting of my decisions, more accepting of myself, far less judgmental of my body, and more able to roll with the punches of life and not use myself as a scapegoat for the inevitable twists and turns that life brings.

In essence, I feel as if I have lived in survival mode for a good part of my life, and I am now just learning how to actually thrive. And I *really* want to thrive. To live out my dreams: I want to become fluent in a second language and live, even temporarily, in a place I where I can speak that language regularly. I want to read more, become a better cook. I want to reach more parents and caregivers on this journey and provide them with even more support than I already do. Perhaps even find a loving partner to share my life with.

But I also live with the reality that the road of loving and advocating for my daughter, V, who lives with emotional and developmental challenges is oftentimes a bumpy one in which I find myself in survival mode. V will need me throughout her life—that is reality.

Along with my ex-husband, I will be her guardian and monitor her finances, medication, therapy, medical decisions, and living arrangements. I will do my best to keep her safe and help her to live her best life.

And with this incredible responsibility, I often ask myself how I can possibly not only survive, but thrive.

As parents and caregivers, our roles often involve being emotional and sometimes physical shock absorbers for our children, fighting for and sometimes with them. But we are also human beings who deserve to live our lives in abundance. To flourish, despite the difficult realities we may live within.

Our journeys to thriving will look and feel different, and that's for everyone, whether or not they are on this path with a child. But for those on this path, we might think of thriving more in terms of "micro moments" that we fit into our daily lives. I often hear of these moments in stories from friends doing their best to thrive, not just survive:

- A friend whose child is on the spectrum and in need of a great deal of daily care and support took a few days to travel and spend with her other child who recently moved to the West Coast. In those days away, my friend stepped over from day-to-day survival to thriving. I loved hearing the lightness of her voice as she described the excitement of waiting at the airport for her flight and the time she spent away.

- After struggling for years and most recently becoming a physical threat to himself and his family, a twelve-year-old child living with mental illness was placed in a residential psychiatric facility. His parents felt a gut-wrenching mixture of guilt, exhaustion, sadness, and ultimately relief that their son was somewhere he could get the help and twenty-four-hour supervision he so desperately needed.

The parents decided to go away for a few days to breathe and recharge. It was impossible for them not to worry about their son, but they knew he was safe. So, with that knowledge, they got in their car and drove to another state, where they stayed in a hotel, took long walks in the mornings, rested, and visited good friends in the area. They felt relieved to be away and laughed at the jokes their friends told them to relieve their tension.

Did they feel guilty being away from their son? For enjoying their time away? For laughing so hard at their friends' jokes that they had to hold their sides? Yes. But they also realized that, at least for now, this was what thriving looked like for them.

- Grandparents raising their three grandchildren—each with emotional and behavioral issues—decided to take the day off and have lunch in a nearby park while their grandchildren were at school. For a few hours, they reconnected and promised themselves that despite the bumpiness of most days, they would regularly take these mini getaways from then on.

- A mother decided to take a once-in-a-lifetime trip to Italy. Her adult son has struggled with mental illness since his late teens and often disappears for weeks at a time, ignoring her calls and pleas to seek help. When he does come home, he is often physically and emotionally abusive toward her. However, with the support of some good friends, she left for her trip abroad. Although she felt conflicted in leaving, she also found many periods of pure joy during her trip and was grateful that she went.

I move from survival mode to thriving when I take time to do things for myself. Things like taking piano lessons, sitting alone in a cafe sipping a delicious cup of coffee as I watch people go by, or striking up conversations with total strangers and perhaps learning something new or even making a friend. (I won't mention my adventures in dating, as lately that has been more survival than anything close to thriving. Oh well . . .)

Here's the thing: I refuse to believe that the rest of our lives will involve various versions of survival, of putting out raging fires or at least bringing them down to a manageable blaze. We all have dreams. Will those dreams need to be adjusted? Yes, and I accept that. It may not be "thriving" in the same way that we imagined or in the way that we see others not on this journey thriving, but I believe we can do more than just survive.

Perhaps as parents and caregivers on this path, we can create our own idea of what it means to live in survival mode while tapping into and living within—even momentarily—thriving mode. Let's use that word I mentioned earlier in this chapter: "surthrival."

Here are some ideas for "surthriving" you might try:

- Plan a day just for yourself during the hours your child is in school or a day program. If you work, then plan a personal day just for you. This is YOUR day, so do exactly what brings you joy! Give yourself a vacation from your personal "to do" list on this day off and just "do you."

- Buy a magazine that covers something of interest to you and take a momentary vacation from life as you flip through its pages.

- Have your favorite snack, and don't share it with anyone.

- Change your environment, even just for a few minutes. Go to a cafe, sit down, and just breathe for a bit. Go to a local library and browse through the bookshelves.

- Make a list of everything you would like to do in your life—and I mean *everything*—no matter the cost, time involved, etc. No one but you needs to see this list. Let your mind run free.

- Give yourself permission *not* to answer phone calls, emails, and texts (even for just a brief period of time).

- Have a good belly laugh. Everyone's sense of humor is different, so find something that makes you laugh. My personal favorites are comic books by Gary Larson, the cable show *Curb Your Enthusiasm*, or watching old episodes of *I Love Lucy*. And if you love Lucy like I do, look up the episode where Lucy and Ethel are working in a chocolate factory. You'll definitely have a good laugh with that one!

From my experiences and those of others on this path, there is a place somewhere between surviving and thriving where parents and caregivers of minor and adult children living with challenges can live, breathe, and grow. A place where laughter and joy live alongside the more difficult emotions we feel on this journey. Where day trips, weekend escapes, and vacations are enjoyed despite the anxiety, guilt, shame, frustration, sadness, and anger. Where our dreams can be lived and realized alongside our fears and restlessness. I realize this may seem impossible given your current reality, but please try, because I promise you are well worth it.

I wish you a happy "surthrival."

Chapter 10 Takeaways

- Parents often feel that they are living in survival mode rather than living life to its fullest.

- Getting out of survival mode may be more difficult for parents and caregivers of children living with challenges, but it is very possible.

- Incorporating small "micro moments" of joy into our lives can help us tap into moments where we are thriving.

- There can be a realistic balance between simply surviving and thriving.

For Further Thought

1. What types of "micro moments" can you create and work into your daily life that will allow you to thrive? (For example: taking a walk, relaxing with a cup of tea, taking time to watch a favorite program without interruption, watching YouTube to explore a particular interest or place in the world, or reading an inspirational passage.) Make a list and look at it often to remind yourself of ways to thrive within your day.

2. What are your favorite types of videos? Most of us have seen video clips—on platforms such as YouTube, Instagram, and TikTok—that bring us momentary joy, excitement, or just good ole

satisfaction. Take a few minutes and escape into your favorite video on a smartphone or other electronic device. Here are a few favorite types of videos friends have shared with me:

- Plane takeoffs and landings (my personal favorite pick-me-up.)

- Anything to do with dogs or cats (There's one video on Instagram of various dogs taking flying leaps into huge piles of leaves that I've watched at least two hundred times and sent to anyone I think needs a video pick-me-up).

- Makeup tutorials
- Cooking videos
- Music videos of favorite songs

Self-Care Workshop – Just Dance

Wherever you are, put on your favorite upbeat song and just dance. I can't tell you how many strange looks I've gotten as I bop along to my favorite tune while stopped at a red light (and I don't care!). Give it a try—you'll be surprised at how good you feel!

Acknowledgments
(and just plain grateful...)

It is impossible to write a book in a vacuum; so many people have helped me bring this book to fruition and I owe them my deepest, most heartfelt thanks.

First and foremost, thank you to the many parents and caregivers who trusted me with their stories and experiences. It is my hope that I have clearly represented your voices for all to hear, learn, and feel connected.

It feels as if I did a million drafts of this book (well, that's overstating it a bit...) I thank all of the readers who so graciously and carefully guided me through the various drafts and provided me with extremely helpful feedback and ideas that made this an even better book than I could have imagined.

A very special thanks to Carol Cohen. Who knew that email you sent me years ago after listening to the podcast would have led to this?! I am forever grateful to have you in my life as a beautiful, calming, and trusted friend on this journey and for your amazing work in helping me run the Sheltered Journey nonprofit organization.

Ilse Wolfe, how much coffee, conversation, laughter, and tears have we shared over the years? Thank you for your never-ending encouragement and for compassionately reminding me of my own words (which I often forget).

Beth Mangiaracina-Ross, what would I do without you dear sister? Thank you for being my memory and for always listening and believing me. An angel was surely by my side in 1988 when I first met you at Family Service of Westchester. You truly are the love of my life.

To my children, sometimes it feels as if we share the same heart. I thank you for your love and encouragement in sharing our stories. I am so proud of you both and stand in absolute respect and awe as I watch you grow into loving, courageous, and resilient women. I will always be your loudest (and, at times, most embarrassing) cheerleader.

Made in the USA
Middletown, DE
24 December 2024